Riding The Waves

Riding The Waves

Diagnosing, Treating, and Living with EMF Sensitivity

Elizabeth Maxim

Published by:
Elizabeth Maxim

ISBN-13: 978-0-61-539546-3
ISBN-10: 0-61-539546-5

1/11

elizabethmaxim.com

With love and thanks to Aaron, my dreamcatcher, who encouraged me to never let go of my dream.

And to Dylan and Hunter, for being my office mates.

CONTENTS

CONTENTS

Acknowledgments

I would like to express my gratitude to the following individuals for their tireless support and assistance with this book: Aaron Maxim, Derek Gauger, Brook Brown, Ken Hutchinson, and Robert Hamaker

I would also like to thank the following people for their friendship and encouragement as I walked the author's path: Mike Trebilcott, Barb and Dick Cole, Maureen Trebilcott, Michael Trebilcott, Anne McKenna, Gregg and Kim Nichols, Tom Keel, Deborah Fruchey, Scott MacKercher, Sue and John Gainey, Andy Wick, Robert Paris, Richard Parker, Jack MacKercher, Tim Barrie, Mary Travis, Dr. Arturo Paz, Dr. Robert Levine, Dr. David Brownstein and the staff at the Center for Holistic Medicine, Dr. John C Webster, Dr. Yuan-da Fan, Dr. Stacia Lansman and the staff at Pediatric Alternatives, RWA, and the Northern Colorado Writers Group

And finally, to Eric Hoheisel, for giving me my first copy of *The Writer's Market* and setting me on the path.

FOREWORD

You have just purchased a book that may very well be the most important health guide in your repertoire. This incredible work provides invaluable insight into a complex and scarcely researched condition as well as beneficial techniques which will extend far beyond traditional methods for improving your physical, emotional, and interpersonal well being.

EMF Sensitivity (Electro Magnetic Frequency Sensitivity) is a commonly misunderstood condition, ironically primarily by the medical community and by those who suffer from it. Most of us recognize that the proliferation of electronic devices in our daily lives has made them not only ubiquitous but also integral to our lifestyles. This holds true regardless of the rate at which any one individual integrates technology in their life. Nearly every electrical device from mobile phones, remote controls, microwave ovens, to household appliances has the potential to emit EMFs in varying degrees of magnitude and in various frequency bands. The pervasiveness of these devices in our daily lives is increasing at an alarming rate and there is nothing that we as individuals can do to abate or avert this. For the few out there who are educated about the detrimental effects of the EMFs, this is an alarming reality; for the vast majority, unaware of this causal relationship, the negative impact of the EMFs on their equilibrium is endured as something "unexplainable," "confusing," and "frustrating."

The engineering community has, for many years, understood the EMF interactions between electrical devices in the context of science. In this community, the terms EMI (electro magnetic interference) and EMC (electro magnetic compatibility) have been well understood and a vast amount of engineering effort has been applied to dealing with the complexities and challenges associated with both. Great effort and time have been expended on engineering and testing in order to make electronic devices compatible with one another; and, extensive studies have been conducted to understand the general environment of the electromagnetic world.

I have explained my condition of EMF Sensitivity to fellow scientists as EMI or Electro Magnetic Intolerance; the concept resonated well with them largely due to our shared engineering background.

Although sophisticated methods of testing and international standards have been developed to guide the engineering community in device-to-device interactions from EMFs, few studies exist for these interactions with humans. The few exceptions are standards that address the extreme case where extraordinarily strong EMFs can cause severe damage to the body such as the development of tumors.

This is precisely why Elizabeth's research is immensely important. It will guide you through the steps of degrading the negative effects and enhancing your "immunity" against the condition.

I truly believe that everyone suffers to some extent from EMF Sensitivity. Some, like myself and Elizabeth, go through a daily struggle ranging from low levels of anxiety to debilitating symptoms. In some of the extreme cases, the symptoms combined with the medical community's lack of understanding, can severely impact one's personal relationships and well-being. When one explores even the most simplistic models of the human body as a system (much like the engineering community would approach a design), they are still faced with a vastly complex and, despite the existing research, a largely misunderstood science. What we do know is that the human body is an intricate electro-chemical system; therefore, it should not be at all surprising that the overabundance of electrical devices in our lives actually do disrupt the system, hence the balance of human health.

For most of us, answering the question of whether or not we have

EMF Sensitivity and to what extent is difficult. Those who are too young to remember the days when computers, cell phones, computer controlled cars, and digital music systems didn't exist, you have never lived in an environment with much lower EMF levels. For those who aren't, the transition both to higher levels and the associated symptoms has been gradual.

I belong to the latter group. It wasn't until I met Elizabeth when I realized that my "habit" of continually "breaking" electronic devices (I can never make a cell phone last more than 8 months) was not just bad fortune; that walking into a room full of computers and feeling anxious was not coincidental; that feeling depressed in an office lit by fluorescent lights was not circumstantial. For those of you who may have a similar condition and are unaware as I was, it requires an open mind to come to terms with it. It's just the same as visiting a doctor's office and being diagnosed with an ailment whose origin and remedy are both foreign.

On a much more positive note, *Riding the Waves* provides all of us with solutions, many of which are not costly or are entirely free of charge. Elizabeth's work is both poignant and pragmatic. I predict sufferers will relate immediately while skeptics will perhaps have difficulty with certain aspects of the book, particularly in the first section where Elizabeth describes many of her extreme case conditions. I encourage all of you to continue reading through to the ensuing sections as I believe that everyone can benefit from understanding EMF Sensitivity. Elizabeth, a well educated, caring, and insightful practitioner, writes from the heart in a grounded manner, much like the way she interacts with patients, friends, and family.

With well wishes for harmony and health, enjoy!

Derek Gauger
CEO, Proxisafe Ltd.

ABOUT THIS BOOK

The material in the following pages may contain information that is the opinion of the author and not necessarily that of your health care provider. It is not intended to replace the advice of a physician. Please consult with your health care provider on specific medical questions.

For continuing updates please check out my website at **www.elizabethmaxim.com**.

PART I

ELIZABETH'S STORY

◊ **ONE** ◊

A Shocking Discovery

JULY 1, 2009
INTERSTATE 580, BAY AREA, CA

"THIS is where I start to feel bad," I said, gazing up at the Oakland Hills.

The San Francisco skyline, visible in the passenger side mirror, receded into the distance.

"This is the Hayward Fault," my husband replied, his hands on the wheel.

"Then it gets better for a bit and then starts up again further up the freeway, at 680."

"That's the Calaveras Fault," he answered.

"Interesting," I responded, absently drumming my fingers against the door. "There aren't any in San Francisco, you know."

I was silent as we drove through the Caldecott Tunnel, mentally reviewing symptoms, dates, and locations. My eyes widened. The fault lines were making me sick.

◊ TWO ◊

A MYSTERY BEGINS

WE relocated to the Bay Area in the fall of 2000 after I received a job transfer. Wanting to get a feel for the different neighborhoods before buying a home, we rented an apartment near my office in the East Bay. Shortly thereafter, I began to experience health issues, the worst of which was severe fatigue. I also had difficulty sleeping and a recurrence in migraines, a problem I hadn't suffered from in years.

At first, I was willing to chalk it up to the stress of moving across the country and starting a new job. However, as time progressed and things settled down but the symptoms didn't, I decided to look deeper. I scheduled a physical.

The doctor and I discussed low thyroid as a possible cause of the fatigue and he ordered the appropriate blood tests. I asked for something to help me sleep, figuring that after about three full nights of sleep, my body's natural rhythm would kick in and I'd be fine.

Most of the physical was routine. However, an EKG turned up an irregularity; inverted T waves. These waves on an EKG represent the resetting of the electrical cells in the bottom chamber of the heart. This was a surprise as previous EKGs had always been normal. The doctor didn't seem overly concerned but still made a note of the new development in my chart. The rest of the physical went well; no health issues were uncovered.

The test results from the blood work showed my thyroid hormone levels within the normal range. However, since I was still suffering from severe fatigue, the doctor prescribed thyroid medication to see if it would make a difference.

After a few weeks I returned for follow up blood work. The fatigue hadn't improved so we began to look for other causes, including low dopamine levels. He suggested I try an anti-depressant. I didn't think I was depressed but if it would help with the fatigue, I was willing to give it a try.

When I returned for the results of the second blood test the doctor told me that my thyroid levels had actually gone down. He explained that my thyroid gland, in response to the supplemental medication, had scaled back production. This was an indication that low thyroid was not the source of the problem. We both agreed that I should stop taking the medication.

A short time after that I quit taking the anti-depressants. I actually felt worse while taking them, and in any event, I didn't feel I was depressed.

Over the next several months I continued to struggle with fatigue, migraines, and difficulty sleeping. I tried natural therapies, including Bach Flower Remedies, vitamins, and juicing, but nothing helped.

In the summer of 2001, we bought a condo in San Francisco. Almost immediately after moving in, the symptoms vanished. I no longer had difficulty sleeping and my energy levels surged. My headaches disappeared and life returned to normal.

We lived in the city for four years until, with our first child eight months old, we decided to purchase a house. After an extensive search, we settled on the East Bay and moved into our home in August 2005.

Soon after moving in I began to feel unwell, lethargic. As the days passed, I realized something was wrong, though I wasn't sure what. At first I said nothing, just tried to organize my thoughts and get a better understanding of what was happening. Unable to point to anything specific and finding no logical explanation, I focused on the mundane tasks associated with settling into a new home and neighborhood.

However, simply ignoring the symptoms didn't make them go away. As the months passed I began to feel worse. I started having difficulty concentrating which took a toll on my writing career. I was tired and run down. I had a sense that things were going in the wrong direction, though I had nothing specific to point to.

My husband, Aaron, listened patiently as I tried, but failed, to find the words to describe what I was going through. He was supportive, but pointed out that we hadn't lived there very long and suggested I give it a little more time; that things may get better. Although this went against my gut feelings, it was certainly a logical approach, so I pushed uncertainty aside in favor of waiting for things to improve.

Unfortunately, as the weeks and months passed, the rundown feeling worsened to a terrible fatigue, and I began to feel depressed about being so tired all the time.

I talked to my doctor but nothing ever turned up; all medical tests came back normal. I followed up with my ob/gyn. All the blood tests he ordered came back normal. Post-natal vitamins especially formulated for extreme fatigue had no noticeable effect. Herbs that strengthened the adrenals were ineffective. I tried acupuncture and Chinese herbs. Any positive effect was very temporary.

In 2006, I became pregnant with our second child. The fatigue was unbelievable. Even the doctor seemed surprised at how tired I was, especially when the fatigue lasted the entire pregnancy.

"Maybe next time you'll feel better," he would say sympathetically.

In addition to the constant exhaustion, I found myself suffering from a mysterious skin irritation on my left wrist and hand. Although the skin looked absolutely normal, no rash or redness, it itched terribly. I removed my watch and scrubbed it. I tried cleansing the skin, but it continued to itch. Thinking it could be dry skin, I tried moisturizer, but that didn't help either. I tried switching laundry detergent and bath soap, changing my diet, but nothing made a difference.

One night, when I couldn't sleep because of the itching. I decided to try Benadryl© lotion. Fortunately, I got enough relief that I was finally able to fall asleep. However, nothing completely eliminated the problem and the symptoms of skin irritation continued to come and go at random for no explicable reason.

◊ THREE ◊

INVESTIGATIONS AND REVELATIONS

AS time went on I became more firmly convinced that whatever was wrong had to do with where we were living. Unfortunately, I didn't know why that might be the case, and I had no proof.

I continued to feel depressed which was truly unusual for me. I lamented that I was too young to feel so old and too healthy to feel so sick.

Traditional medical tests always came back normal and my physicals, aside from the inverted T waves, hadn't turned anything up. Since I have a doctorate in holistic medicine, I left no stone unturned in considering alternate remedies. I pursued every natural therapy I could think of. Unfortunately, nothing seemed to help.

Then, starting in April 2008, I noticed that periodically the fatigue would become so severe that I was practically debilitated. It got to the point where I refused to drive on those days because I felt my ability to react was impaired; that I couldn't drive safely. My eyes burned with fatigue and I felt heaviness in the area of my forehead. Everything seemed to slow down and I had difficulty concentrating. It was as if someone had poured molasses on my brain.

I never knew when this extreme fatigue would hit. It would last approximately three days and then improve to the constant level of fatigue that I struggled with on a daily basis.

I continued to feel very depressed. In fact, I'd noticed that at times, the depression darkened to a feeling of hopelessness and deep despair. I was completely puzzled by these symptoms because there didn't seem to be any logical explanation for them. Strangely, the depression was kind of hollow; it didn't feel emotionally or mentally created. I began to wonder if the constant fatigue was making me feel depressed or if I really *was* depressed and one of the symptoms was constant fatigue. What was truly puzzling, however, was the fact that the feelings of depression would come and go, seemingly at random, for no identifiable reason.

Interestingly, although I felt these overwhelmingly dark moods come over me; I never felt they were part of me. As crazy as it sounded, I continued to insist that whatever was happening was not psychological, emotional, or mental. I knew something very wrong was happening. I didn't have an explanation for it and I had no cause I could point to, but I knew myself. I knew that whatever was going on was outside of me; that I was reacting to something. I knew it in my gut.

Still, I believed a bit of due diligence was in order. I contacted my father and a couple of longtime friends to discuss my disposition. All of them agreed that I was generally an upbeat person not prone to depression, and that I was someone who rebounded rather quickly from the curve balls life occasionally threw. I certainly felt vindicated by their assurances, but also frustrated. I still had no explanation for the mysterious symptoms.

It was at this same time, April 2008, that I began to suffer a constant runny nose, mucous drainage, and my eyes would water and burn.

What next?!

Resenting this new development, I tried allergy medication but got little relief. I tried cold tablets but that didn't work at all. I switched back to allergy medication, trying a different brand. I got some relief, but not much.

I was still having the itching problem on my left wrist and hand, but I was fairly certain it was not an allergic reaction. There were no visible signs of irritation; no rash, no redness, and no swelling. Additionally, it came and went at random, not in response to any specific event or stimuli.

I read up on allergies and although severe fatigue was listed as a symptom, I wasn't convinced. My instincts told me that my symptoms were being caused by something other than a simple allergy. Besides, if it was an allergy, why wouldn't it have started right after we moved into our house, back in 2005?

Interestingly, I had noticed that when we were away from home, I often felt better. This suggested that whatever was causing the issue was very close to the house, so, in spite of my strong belief that the symptoms were not the result of an allergic reaction, I did some intense detective work.

To start, I considered any changes I might have made, including detergents, food and beverage choices, lifestyle changes, anything I thought could result in the strange symptoms.

Next, I considered the trees and plants in our neighborhood. With the exception of the sycamores and the Monterey pines, I had been around most of them at other times in my life and never recalled having had a problem. In fact, I had never before suffered allergy symptoms like the ones that began in April 2008.

Withholding judgment, I went about normal activities, always paying close attention to when and where I felt better or worse. One day we took the kids to a nearby park and I noticed that in spite of the fact that we were surrounded by the same trees and plants that grew near our home, my symptoms were absent. Obviously, I could put the allergy theory to rest.

Life continued to be punctuated by symptoms that varied in severity, that would come and go, seemingly at random. This made getting to the bottom of what was going on a supreme challenge. Then, one summer day in 2009, a casual conversation with Aaron changed everything.

We lived in the Bay Area. The implications that fault lines were compromising my health were staggering.

◊ FOUR ◊

TESTING THE THEORY

IF fault lines were in fact making me sick then I should feel the symptoms, not just in the East Bay, but anywhere where they were located.

I discussed the situation with a friend who is a mechanical engineer. It was gratifying to be able to talk about the issue in-depth with an objective third party. Derek not only agreed my hypothesis had merit, he suggested it would be easy enough to test. As we sat eating lunch at the *Sea Breeze* in Berkeley, he outlined his idea to both Aaron and I. Aaron would create a driving route that would take us over and near various fault zones around the Bay Area. As a passenger, I would make note of any symptoms or lack of them and see if they coincided with the location of those fault lines. Naturally, I would have to be unaware of the location of any fault lines Aaron selected. This would prove to be an easy requirement to fulfill.

As a transplant, my knowledge of Bay Area faults was pretty limited. Other than what I'd learned decades before in a geology 101 course, my only understanding was that the Hayward Fault was probably in Hayward, the Calaveras Fault was near Pleasanton, and the San Andreas Fault was somewhere out in the Pacific Floor. Complying with the conditions of the test would be simple.

Aaron obtained fault line data from the United States Geological Survey (USGS)[1]. Their website soon became a valuable resource in our efforts to get to the bottom of what was happening.

He mapped out a route for our first test. Armed with a notebook, we packed the family into the car. I took my place in the passenger seat and we set out to see if we could confirm my suspicions.

I scribbled out information, noting symptoms, their severity, and the locations where I was affected. I also wrote down when and where they eased up. The symptoms came and went pretty instantaneously, as if someone was flipping a switch on and off.

About halfway through the trip Aaron told me it was evident I was able to correctly identify the locations of fault lines based on feedback I gave him about how I was feeling. The symptoms coincided with fault locations on the route he'd designed.

At one point we passed through an area where Route 4 veered toward the city of Richmond. I felt symptoms quite intensely, yet Aaron said he wasn't aware of any fault lines nearby; none had shown on the map he'd referenced. I countered by pointing out that the maps would only list known fault lines, and that more than once authorities had become aware of a fault line only after an earthquake alerted them to its existence.

I was able to subsequently confirm the presence of a fault line in that exact location when the USGS reported a quake on it only a week later.

The drive around the Bay Area was certainly illuminating. By the time we'd returned home I was exhausted. I felt as if I'd been beat up. For several miles and for over an hour I had experienced one or more symptoms, including difficulty breathing, dizziness, a runny nose, burning, watery eyes, mucous drainage in my throat, a tightness in my chest, a knot in my stomach, nausea, and heartburn, something I'd never suffered from in my life.

Symptoms turned on and off in a very precise way. The moment we were on or very close to a fault line, they appeared. Once we'd moved on, they vanished as if they were never there.

The experiment was indeed a success. The fault lines were definitely making me sick.

The question was, why?

◊ FIVE ◊

THE RESEARCH

MY initial research into the geology of our planet proved fruitful in that I learned a great deal about fault lines. Unfortunately, none of it explained why I was feeling so sick around them. Obviously, more investigation was needed.

Even as I dreaded the prospect of feeling so awful, I needed to learn more, so, more driving was in order. Aaron chauffeured me around, varying the route but always making sure to travel near and over fault lines, which isn't difficult when you live in the San Francisco Bay Area.

It made sense to be chauffeured for these experiments for a number of reasons. For one, I was able to take notes in a spiral notebook I was keeping for that purpose. Secondly, I had someone who could act as a witness and assistant. Lastly, because the symptoms were debilitating at times, it was better to have a healthy person behind the wheel.

◊ ◊ ◊ ◊ ◊

"Do you think it could be electromagnetic waves?" I wondered aloud as my family drove back from Berkeley one afternoon.

It certainly seemed plausible to me that waves from the earth's magnetic core could travel up through the fault lines, through the atmosphere, and into my cells where they proceeded to wreak havoc. But how could I test such a hypothesis?

At that point I had to smile at one of life's little ironies. I had married an electrical engineer. Who better to discuss the principles of electromagnetic theory with?

Aaron and I had an in-depth discussion about electromagnetic waves including the highly flammable debate regarding whether or not electromagnetic frequencies (EMFs) were harmful to humans.

"I wouldn't be surprised if electromagnetic waves came out of the fault lines," Aaron answered. "That's an opening in the earth. I'm just not sure what part of the spectrum that would be."

The electromagnetic (EM) spectrum is the name used to refer to various types of wave-based radiation; radiation being energy that travels and spreads out as it goes. The different types of energy on the spectrum are described in terms of wavelength, and amplitude. Amplitude is the magnitude of the wave. Wavelength is the distance from the top of one wave to the next. Frequency is the number of waves passing a point per second, measured in Hertz (Hz).

Radio, microwave, infrared, ultraviolet, X-rays, and Gamma-rays are all forms of electromagnetic energy and refer to ranges of frequency. They appear on the spectrum in order from lowest to highest and because wavelength is inversely proportional to its frequency, energies with the lowest frequencies have the longest wavelengths. This means they can travel the furthest distance and, surprisingly, may have the strongest impact.

It's understood that the energies at the high end of the frequency spectrum are highly radioactive and pose a threat to human health, but what about those at the opposite end?

"I worked in the technology industry for nearly twenty years and never had any issues," I pointed out. "I've never had any problems around cell phones or microwaves either; at least, none that I'm aware of."

I paused, thinking. I needed to prove whether or not electromagnetic waves were causing the symptoms, but how?

As we drove through the Caldecott tunnel I thought about the nature of electromagnetic waves. If I could find something to absorb the waves in place of my cells or at least deflect them away from my body, and I got relief from the symptoms, I could be pretty sure I had my answer. So, what could I use?

"Too bad I don't have a Faraday cage."

Also known as a Faraday shield, the device is an enclosure used to block external static electrical fields, and, if constructed for such a purpose, electromagnetic radiation[2]. Anything and anyone inside such a device would be protected.

However, since I couldn't get my hands on such a device, nor easily build one in my backyard, I knew I had to focus on materials I could get access to.

"I wonder if lodestone would help, or quartz crystal?"

Touted by New Age practitioners for their therapeutic and grounding properties, crystals and minerals have a history in healing that spans multiple cultures and goes back thousands of years. In fact, I had studied these modalities while earning my doctorate; with a course in vibrational medicine and one in magnetic healing. While my family waited in the car, I paid a visit to a local New Age store.

I easily found the section with baskets full of minerals, crystals, and stones purported to heal or otherwise promote well-being. Excited, I reached for a large piece of lodestone, a naturally magnetized piece of the mineral magnetite, fairly certain that once I held it I would feel a moment of *Ahh*.

To my utter dismay, a strong burning electrical sensation traveled through the fingers of my right hand, up my arm, down my spine and straight down my right leg. Yelping in pain, my arm jerked and I tossed the lodestone away from me. Vigorously shaking out my fingers and leg, I worked to regain my equilibrium. I wiped my hand against my jeans several times before staring at the seemingly innocuous mineral. I had handled lodestone before, while living in San Francisco, and had never had that reaction. I decided to try again. This time, when the same thing happened, I was somewhat prepared, and therefore, a bit more controlled in releasing the stone. I tried holding it in my left hand and although it wasn't quite as painful, I got the same end result.

I picked up an information placard that listed the geologic and reputed healing properties for various crystals and stones, scanning for any others that were magnetic. Tiger iron, a combination of golden tiger's eye, red jasper, and black hematite, was described as having magnetic properties. However, the basket for tiger iron was empty.

I decided to test each stone individually and then collectively by holding all three at once. My lips curled in distaste, however, as I eyed the hematite. Although reputed for grounding and healing properties, I had never been able to touch the stone without feeling immense discomfort. In fact, the sensations I felt when I held the stone were so unpleasant, I decided to forgo including it in my little experiment.

I picked up the golden tiger's eye but felt nothing. Putting it back, I reached for the red jasper. An unpleasant electrical sensation began to move up my arm so I quickly put it back. Although this bit of research had only taken a few minutes, I had gained a great deal of knowledge.

I started to leave when I remembered the quartz crystal. The store had several varieties to choose from, including rose and smoky. However, holding these crystals had absolutely no effect. Putting them back in the baskets, I returned to the car to give my report to Aaron.

◊ SIX ◊

SHINING ARMOR

ONCE we were home, both of us got on the Internet. I kept thinking back to the Faraday cage and my desire to have something absorb the energy in place of my cells.

"I wonder if copper would do the trick?"

I knew from my days working with computer networks that it was an excellent and affordable conduit. Across the room, Aaron nodded and we proceeded to have an in-depth discussion about the conductivity of metals. He located a table that ranked various metals (see *Table 1*). The higher the conductivity was, the better the metal's ability to shield from electromagnetic fields.

Table 1: Sample of Metal Properties

Conductive Materials	Electrical Conductivity (10^6 Siemens/m)	Electrical Resistivity (10^8 Ohm.m)	Thermal Conductivity (W/m.k)
Silver	62.1	1.6	420
Copper	58.5	1.7	401
Gold	44.2	2.3	317
Aluminium	36.9	2.7	237
Zinc	16.6	6.0	116
Brass	15.9	6.3	150
Nickel	14.3	7.0	91
Lithium	10.8	9.3	85
Iron	10.1	9.9	80
Palladium	9.5	10.5	72
Platinium	9.3	10.8	107
Tungsten	8.9	11.2	174
Tin	8.7	11.5	67
Bronze (67%Cu/33%Zn)	7.4	13.5	85
Carbon steel	5.9	16.9	90
Lead	4.7	21.3	35
Titanium	2.4	41.7	21
Stainless Steel (316L)	1.8	55.6	15
Mercury	1.1	90.9	8

Source: Tibtech Innovations

I noted that copper was second only to silver when it came to shielding strength.

"Silver is ideal but it's too expensive," Aaron pointed out. "That's why copper is used in homes and office buildings."

In fact, copper is the de facto standard for conductive material.

I noticed that stainless steel was toward the bottom of the list. I stared at my watch, considering. Since moving to California I had had to replace the battery two to three times more often than average. I even had one jeweler jokingly suggest that I offer my services to battery manufacturers as a tester.

Staring at the stainless steel band, I pursed my lips. Even if my watch was absorbing some of the waves in place of my cells, it wasn't effective enough to lessen the negative physical effects.

"I found the frequency of fault lines," Aaron called from across the room.

I gave him my attention.

"Wow, it's really low. It's something like .01 Hz."

I didn't know much about the ultra-low frequencies on the electromagnetic spectrum other than that they traveled farther distances than their higher counterparts.

"I remember reading in that book, *The Intention Experiments,* that researchers had had a hard time shielding some of the experiments from magnetic waves," I told him. "They used a Faraday cage. I really want to try the copper."

Fortunately, my kids love a trip to the hardware store almost as much as a trip to the toy store. While they played with little plastic gizmos and gadgets I grabbed onto a rope of copper wrapped around a spool.

"Nothing," I said, disappointed. My plan had been to buy some of the copper and fashion it into a bracelet or necklace and see how that worked.

"Maybe you should go try that jewelry?" Aaron suggested, referring to copper bracelets sold at golf supply and New Age stores. They had a reputation for healing.

With nothing to lose, I went back to the New Age store. Idly, I wondered if they were thinking, *Oh no, here's that lady again. I hope she doesn't throw anything this time.*

On the counter was a selection of bracelets. Although some of them were purely copper, most of the ones displayed were a combination of copper, silver, and jeweler's brass. I tried one made from copper only and felt nothing.

I then selected a pretty one with all three metals fashioned in a wave-like design. The moment I placed it on my right wrist I felt an immediate sense of relief and a slight, though not painful, tingling on my arm. Excited, I wondered if the effect was cumulative. I added a second bracelet, also made of all three metals, and felt even better.

Since I already had my watch with the stainless steel band on my left wrist, I decided that a single bracelet would probably be sufficient. Through trial and error I decided that one made from copper and silver felt best. Ecstatic at the relief I felt, not to mention the surge of energy, I purchased the bracelets and drove home, anxious to share the good news with Aaron.

I'd found a cure.

Or, so I thought.

◊ SEVEN ◊

STORMY SEAS

IT seemed too fantastical that just wearing bracelets made of copper, silver, and brass could have such a profound effect on my health, but I couldn't argue with how much better I felt. I had more energy than I'd had in years, the itching on my left wrist and hand had stopped and the allergy symptoms I'd been suffering from for over a year had vanished completely. I no longer had a runny nose or watery, burning eyes. I was thrilled that my theory had proven valid and that there was even a scientific explanation.

Magnetic shielding is achieved when materials are used to create an area of higher magnetic field. Essentially, the bracelets, with their higher magnetic field, were drawing the waves, absorbing them in place of my cells, just as I'd theorized.

Still, further testing was needed. I wanted to know, for instance, if anything else would have the same effect. Salt water, perhaps?

I loved the ocean. I felt energized sitting on a beach, smelling the salty air, and watching the waves roll in. I had read something about negative ions improving human health but felt it rather inconclusive. Still, there was something healing about salt water.

That evening I removed the bracelets and got into a bath into which I'd added a cup of baking soda and a half a cup of non-iodized sea salt. I chose this combination not only because of the salinity it would create but also because it is a healing bath in and of itself.

Within minutes of removing the bracelets I began to feel poorly. I paid attention to the symptoms and their severity and decided that, in the bath, they weren't quite as bad. I suspected this was because of the salt content of water. I believed it was acting as a low-level shielding. After I got out of the bath I put the bracelets back on. Within minutes I was feeling better.

My next test was to drive back over the fault zones while wearing the bracelets and see if I noticed any difference. This time I drove alone. I discovered new areas where I felt symptoms and noted that, although I was still able to feel the physical effects when I was on or very close to fault lines, the symptoms didn't seem to be quite as severe and there weren't as many of them. The bracelets were definitely working.

The medical use of copper dates back to ancient Egypt and Rome[3]. Early theories suggested that copper worn next to the skin was absorbed into the bloodstream through the dermis, facilitating healing.

I had noticed that there was a unique green coloring on my wrists, and that the veins near where the bracelets touched my skin had raised closer to the surface, appearing to be almost engorged.

That evening I checked my husband's wrist. He had purchased a bracelet made from silver and brass. While his reaction wasn't as strong as mine, he said he noticed a slight tingling sensation, adding that he felt the bracelet had a soothing effect.

Sure enough, the veins near the bracelet were close to the surface and very green. He also had the same slight discoloration on his skin.

I didn't believe this was the discoloration some people got when they wore cheap jewelry; a result of a chemical reaction. I had never had such a reaction to any jewelry. The green hue near where the bracelets touched our skin did not wash off, and it faded and reappeared at random.

Anxious to get my mind off my symptoms, we decided to do something fun. We decided to go hiking. Of course, since fault zones and mountains go together like peas and carrots, I knew this meant being subjected to some physical discomfort. However, my life had become a living experiment anyway, so I chose to focus on learning everything I could while doing something I loved. Besides, I had the bracelets.

We hiked at a vigorous pace and both of us carried the extra weight of a child. However, since I exercised regularly and was physically fit, I was only slightly winded. In fact, I realized that I had more difficulty breathing when simply sitting in the car near a fault line than from hiking up a mountain, carrying a toddler in the extreme heat associated with East Bay summers.

As we hiked back down at a vigorous pace, I realized that the stress response from my body was significantly different when breathless from exercise than when breathless from exposure to fault lines. It certainly seemed that my adrenals were far less stressed from mere exercise.

The days progressed and I continued to monitor symptoms, their severity, the location they were felt, and anything else I considered relevant. Heat, for instance.

A few days got into triple digits Fahrenheit and Aaron pointed out that I seemed to feel worse when the temperature spiked. I tried to learn if there was a relationship between heat and magnetic waves, but was unable to find anything conclusive. The best I could do was to monitor my own body and see if the higher temperatures consistently magnified the symptoms.

Between keeping a journal of what was happening, transcribing notes, exchanging emails, and doing online research, I was spending a great deal of time at my computer. Even as I was typing, clicking, and emailing, one part of my mind was

34

always on the symptoms I was experiencing. It was because of this that I noticed another significant detail. My symptoms worsened cyclically. In fact, they kept business hours.

◊ EIGHT ◊

GETTING OUT OF DODGE

I TYPICALLY got on the computer around eight in the morning. Beginning around nine I would start to have difficulty breathing. By eleven thirty, a low level dizziness set in. The symptoms would increase in severity, peaking somewhere around four in the afternoon, and sharply reducing between five and seven in the evening. By the time I crawled into bed at night, I was completely exhausted, though my symptoms were not nearly as bad.

I needed to understand more about this strange pattern; whether or not it was consistent on weekends and whether or not it existed if I was out of the area. It was time to get out of Dodge.

We took off on the first of what would be a series of impromptu research trips. This one would take us to Lake Tahoe, on the California - Nevada border.

During the drive up we went through areas where the symptoms were extremely intense, and areas where I barely noticed anything. Google searches on my cell phone confirmed that the symptoms appeared in the presence of geologic fault lines.

As we checked into our hotel, I realized that I was in for a long weekend. It was obvious by how I was feeling that we were very close to a fault line. I knew my family had hoped I would be able to relax and experience some extended relief, so I said nothing and prepared to make the best of our mini vacation.

While driving toward Carson City the next morning, I noted with great interest that after rounding a bend in the Sierra Nevada Mountain Range my symptoms suddenly and completely vanished. I was puzzled because I had discovered, while researching the Tahoe area the night before, that there were fault lines all over the place. We stopped for gas in Carson City and I continued to notice how really good I felt.

When we drove through Silver City, Nevada, I became aware of a strong electrical sensation surging through my body, and my hands and fingers tingled.

"This town is haunted," I blurted. "I can feel it."

The sensation disappeared once we got into the next city, Gold Hill. We drove further, arriving in Virginia City, but decided to circle back and see if the same sensations presented themselves. Although I didn't experience anything in Gold Hill, once back in Silver City, my hands and fingers tingled, and I felt as if a low level electrical current was surging through me.

"I know this place is haunted," I asserted as we drove back toward Virginia City, where we decided to stop and spend some time.

I enjoyed walking around the old west town. It was the first time in quite awhile that I actually felt good. In fact, I felt so completely normal that I couldn't help but wonder if I had imagined the whole thing.

Had I really felt as bad as I remembered or was memory distorting the severity? More than that, I questioned the source of the problem. Can fault lines make someone ill? Wouldn't I have heard about something like that?

Aaron reminded me of all the research I'd done and assured me that the symptoms were not in my head. Something was definitely happening and the evidence overwhelmingly pointed at fault lines.

I spotted a couple of tourist shops that sold minerals and rocks; one on each side of the street. I decided to go in and see if I got any symptoms. Not long after I entered the first shop I began to feel poorly. I had difficulty breathing and felt very dizzy. When I approached rocks that had magnetic properties, the symptoms worsened. Determined to continue the experiment, I stayed, touching various stones and crystals, noting whether or not I felt better, worse, or no change.

I approached a display of salt lamps and a variety of salt crystals to go with them. Salt lamps are chunks of mined salt that are hollowed out to accommodate a light bulb and salt crystals. While they make an attractive light, they are best known for their reputed health benefits. When the salt crystals are heated they release negative ions into the atmosphere. Negative ions are associated with a reduction in fatigue and other general health improvements.

I touched the round salt crystals and noticed an immediate reduction in symptom severity. This was consistent with my reaction in the salt bath and backed up my theory that salt provided a low-level shielding from the negative effects of the fault lines. Considering the exercise a success, I left the first shop.

It wasn't until I was back outside, standing on the old wooden sidewalk that I realized just how awful I'd been feeling in the shop. I gulped air and enjoyed the absence of symptoms.

While in the store my chest had felt constricted, as if an elephant had been sitting on it. This had affected my ability to breathe normally. I had experienced a strong, almost claustrophobic feeling of oppression. Interestingly, I had also become aware of a new symptom.

While I was in the shop I'd felt as if I had a fever and my skin was unusually warm. I theorized it was because my body was trying to fight the invisible intruder much the same way it would attack a virus, by heating up. Now, out on the sidewalk, I felt much more comfortable; ironic, given it was summer in the Nevada desert.

I looked across the street and caught site of the other shop. Sighing, I shook my head and started across the road. I had to go inside to see if the same thing happened.

Just as in the first store, within a few minutes of entering the shop I began to feel poorly. Since the stones seemed to be the same type sold at the other location, I didn't bother to stick around. I went back out to the sidewalk and took deep breaths, grateful to again be free of symptoms.

Over lunch we talked about the charm of the former mining town, impressed by the historical detail that was so well preserved. However, my mind was, as usual, focused on whether or not I was experiencing any symptoms and how bad they were. It was a bit of a letdown that the situation constantly invaded my thoughts. Although I wanted to learn and understand as much as I could, I was also determined not to let it take over my life.

We drove back toward Tahoe and as we got into Silver City, I again felt an energy surge along with a tingling sensation in my hands. We pulled over so I could get a look around. As I stood next to the car, I pointed toward a large boulder.

"Whatever's causing this, it's coming from there."

My husband glanced over. "It looks like a historical marker."

Without hesitation, I replied, "It's a grave."

What makes that an interesting response is that I had never been to Silver City. I knew absolutely nothing about it or the surrounding area.

Curious, I proceeded to walk around the downtown area. Unlike Virginia City, there wasn't much left of this small town outside a few buildings and the foundations where others had once stood. I paid attention to every bodily sensation, looking for clues. Finally, with my fingers and hands tingling, I approached what I believed to be the source of the strong electrical sensation; a boulder. I read the historical plaque attached to its surface. Shaking my head in disbelief, I returned to the car.

"I was right," I said, buckling my seatbelt. "It's a grave marker."

As we continued out of town, I stared at my hands. They were no longer tingling.

◊ NINE ◊

THE SILVER LINING

BY the time we were back at our hotel in Tahoe I was again experiencing distressing symptoms. I was frustrated at the injustice of having felt so good, only to find myself feeling badly again for no reason I could understand. At this point I decided to share the truth of how badly I'd been feeling while in Tahoe. Although naturally disappointed, Aaron agreed that the absence of symptoms in Nevada, a place so geographically close, not to mention geologically similar, warranted further investigation.

We decided to drive home by driving back through Nevada, which would allow me to assess symptoms along a new route. It would also take us past the areas we had visited the day before.

Before we even reached Carson City I knew there was something special about the area. I not only experienced an absence of symptoms, I actually felt great. I had a surge of energy and a mental clarity I hadn't experienced in a long time. What was it about that area?

"I'm guessing it has to do with the mineral content in the ground here," Aaron stated. "It must be different."

As we drove through the mountains I studied rock surfaces, noting the variety of colors layered throughout. In addition to deep reds, there was quite a bit of green.

"If I didn't know any better, I'd say there was copper in these mountains."

That made no sense to me. I knew there had been silver and gold in the area, but copper? I took out my cell phone and did a Google search.

"You aren't going to believe this," I said, staring at the phone screen in shock. "Not only is there copper in these mountains, but silver and zinc as well."

I stared at my bracelets. Jeweler's brass was an alloy of copper and zinc.

"No wonder I've been feeling so good. I've been standing on the same materials the bracelets are made out of."

I glanced at my wrists. The green discoloration that had been there only that morning, while we were at Lake Tahoe, was gone and my veins had returned to normal size. It was as if my body was getting enough copper from the environment, along with silver and zinc, and didn't need to absorb as much from the bracelets.

Back at home I went straight to the computer, anxious to follow the new lead. I spent hours on the USGS website, first reading up on soil samples to see if there were any differences between Nevada and the Bay Area. The geology of the two states, especially in this geography, was so similar, any differences, I decided, could be discounted. It was definitely looking as if Aaron's theory was correct; the presence of specific minerals in the ground made the difference.

I widened my search to cover the entire state of California, paying attention to areas I believed relevant. The hypothesis held up. The locations I always felt really good in were consistently near old mines; specifically, silver and copper mines. It seemed another field trip was in order.

I decided the quickest way to accomplish the research would be to try a location close enough for a day trip. The answer? Copperopolis, California.

The route we took, CA-4, unfortunately runs near a fault zone. I suffered dizziness, nausea, difficulty breathing, mucous drainage in my throat, burning eyes, and the feeling of being squeezed too tightly.

As we neared the city of Copperopolis, we noticed a significant change in the landscape near the intersection of Telegraph Drive and CA-4. On the west side of the intersection, the landscape was primarily agricultural fields, whereas on the east side there were numerous trees. I also noticed, to my relief, that almost immediately after we drove through the intersection,

45

my symptoms vanished. No sooner had I updated Aaron than we saw outcroppings of rocks bearing the telltale green coloring. Copper.

"Amazing," he muttered.

I talked about the immense relief I was experiencing; particularly from the sensation of being squeezed too tightly. The pressure on my chest during those episodes was extremely unpleasant. Combined with the difficulty breathing, it created a most unwelcome situation and actually caused another, most annoying symptom; yawning.

The depressed respiratory function left me repeatedly trying to gulp air. This continued until I would sigh deeply and then the cycle would start all over again until we got far enough away from the fault zones that I was no longer affected. When away from the fault lines I had no difficulty breathing.

Along with taking deep breaths, I was yawning; constantly. It wasn't your average yawn, either. My head would tilt down and to the right so that my jaw was in the crook of my shoulder. Even as my mouth would begin to widen, my head would jerk in a spasm and before the yawn could complete, my jaw would slam shut. This was not only incredibly frustrating, it was painful, since my body was attempting to yawn every thirty seconds to two minutes. Along with the constant attempt to yawn, my eyes watered and burned.

My initial hypothesis was that the yawns were my body's attempt to compensate for the perceived lack of oxygen caused by depressed respiratory function. However, as I thought about it, it occurred to me that I had been through this once before, some thirty years prior.

When I was a child I had to take the prescription drug Dilantin for a short time. Dilantin is a drug that regulates the electrical activity of brain waves in order to prevent seizures. I had never suffered from epilepsy; I was given the medication as a preventative measure after neurosurgery. One of the side effects I had experienced while taking Dilantin was a type of respiratory distress that caused a frequent, not to mention annoying need to take deep breaths, eventually ending in a sigh. A consequence of this constant need for deep breaths was frequent yawning.

I currently take no medication and had stopped taking the Dilantin decades before. Even so, my body was going through the same traumatic experience, suggesting that my brain waves were being affected in much the same way as when I had been taking the antiepileptic drug. Anxious as I was to learn more about this new detail, I had another experiment to complete first. Next stop, Copperopolis.

Our visit was relatively short. We spent some time downtown and visited Copper Park where mining implements were on display. Having successfully validated the relationship between copper in the ground and insulation from the effects of fault lines, we headed for home. Before leaving, I followed up on a hunch and gathered a few rock samples from the side of the road. I wanted to see if they would make a difference in the symptoms I felt on the return trip.

I collected five rocks total; four small and one larger, heavier one. When the symptoms began, pretty much as we entered the intersection of CA-4 and Telegraph Drive, I picked up a smaller stone. I felt no relief. I held all four smaller stones but still felt no relief. I held the larger greenish rock and within seconds the difficulty breathing all but disappeared, along with the tight feeling in my chest and the dizziness. While this was a wonderful discovery, it presented a bit of a problem. Holding the rock for the long journey home would be daunting; it was heavy. Remembering the statement I'd made days before about standing on the same materials that the bracelets were made of, I put the rock on the floor and rested my feet on its surface. Even through my sneakers the effect was almost immediate. Mercifully, our return trip proved to be much more comfortable.

◊ TEN ◊

PSYCHOBABBLE

UNFORTUNATELY, the reprieve was all too brief. Soon after we got home, the symptoms suddenly and inexplicably worsened as I stood in our front yard. In addition to a very difficult time catching my breath and tightness in my chest, I had a strong sensation that I was dying. The symptoms accelerated, bringing a feeling of panic I believe was the fight or flight response[4].

The severity of the symptoms rarely led to the level of panic I experienced that evening. Even so, I knew I had to find a way to recognize when they were worsening so I could talk my way out of panic before it began. More importantly, I needed to find a way to counter what was causing it in the first place. Obviously, as helpful as the bracelets were, they weren't enough.

Completely worn out from what had happened, I retreated to my office. I placed the four smaller rocks on my desk near my keyboard and the larger one underneath. Resting my feet on it, I launched Google.

Copper obviously made a positive difference but short of walking around in a suit of copper armor or spending my life inside a Faraday cage, I felt there was only so much it could do. Still, I was determined to find consistent relief. I wondered about nutritional supplements. Would taking copper internally help shore up my defense?

I read up on the benefits of copper supplements, astonished by what I discovered. Copper is necessary for energy and respiratory function[5]. Two of the worst symptoms I experienced regularly were severe fatigue and difficulty breathing. Was exposure to the frequencies emitted by fault lines causing a nutritional deficiency? I decided to try mineral supplementation and see if it would make a difference.

That night, as I lay in bed, breathing more easily, I thought over everything that I'd learned, ruthlessly analyzing every detail.

"I just don't understand. I feel completely fine now. It's as if there's nothing wrong with me." I sighed. "This is making me crazy."

"You are not crazy," Aaron assured. "I was there; I saw everything. This is happening to you. It's not in your head. You are not making it up."

"Thanks," I answered quietly. Exhausted, I fell asleep.

The next morning I woke more determined than ever to understand what seemed to be a cyclical relationship to the symptoms. I doubted Mother Nature kept business hours and in any event, when I was away from home, there was no time-related pattern. That suggested that something else was having a negative effect on my body.

"Could it be the wireless?" Aaron asked, indicating the networking equipment located close to my work area.

"I doubt it," I responded. "I spent decades working in technology, constantly around computers and networks, installing them myself, and to my knowledge, nothing ever bothered me. Not to mention, this stuff didn't bother me when we lived in San Francisco."

"I don't know," he persisted. "That's an awful lot of stuff in there. Look, the cordless phone base is in there too."

He volunteered to relocate the equipment but I asked him to hold off. Something told me the wireless equipment was not the problem. I had to dig deeper.

That evening, while reading a book in bed, I again took stock of how I felt.

"You know, you might be right about the wireless equipment. I feel fine here in the bedroom, no difficulty breathing, no symptoms, and there's nothing in here but furniture, a couple of lamps, and a battery operated alarm clock."

He agreed and again suggested we relocate the equipment away from my office.

"Let's wait," I countered. "I want to do more experiments."

The next morning I woke up and went to the living room instead of my office. It's a room I'd always felt good in and, probably not coincidentally, a room I'd decorated with copper accents several years before. It would seem that on some level I had been aware of the situation and had been making attempts to insulate myself.

Sitting down with a book, I looked forward to a morning and possibly an entire day free of symptoms. Unfortunately, right on schedule, the difficulty breathing began.

A couple of days later I was standing in the kitchen talking on one of the cordless phones with a friend. As we were chatting I realized I felt fine where I was. This friend is also an electrical engineer and we had been discussing possible variables, so when I noted the change, we began to discuss it in detail.

"It makes no sense," I maintained. "There are appliances in here, including a microwave." I turned and looked at where my kids were watching TV in the family room. I rarely entered that room. There was a wireless music device in there.

"I guess it could be the wireless," I conceded, though I didn't really believe it. "There's wireless in my office and in the family room, but none in the bedrooms, living room, or dining room. I don't think I have a problem in any of those rooms."

That night I lay in bed, my mind whirling. It seemed that every time I answered one question, two more popped up in its place. Even though the evidence was pointing at wireless equipment, my instinct told me that wasn't what was causing the cyclical effect. As I drifted off to sleep, I made a decision.

It was time to play the detective instead of the scientist.

◇ ELEVEN ◇

YOU ARE NOT CRAZY

ONE of the more disturbing aspects of what was happening to me was the incredible stress my mind and body were under. My brainwaves were being hijacked by EM frequencies and I was helpless to stop it. My autonomic nervous system was being impacted, my ability to think clearly impaired, and my emotions were yo-yoing up and down relative to the severity of the symptoms.

The bracelets I wore helped lessen the intensity of the symptoms but they didn't eliminate them entirely. In fact, there were times when, unexpectedly and inexplicably, the beneficial effect was significantly reduced. I hypothesized this was because there were circumstances when, for whatever reason, EMF levels were higher.

I switched my focus from trying to understand the cause and effect relationship to trying to survive the impact.

I knew that there was only so much I could do to redirect the waves away from my body so I analyzed the nature of energy waves, considering what other options I had. Would it be possible to cancel them out with another type of energy wave? Say, with music?

As I considered the idea further, I became more convinced that music would make a positive difference. After all, sound energy had been used in healing for centuries and I had personal experience observing the effects of music on my health.

I knew, for instance, that as far back as high school, I was aware that certain songs left me feeling depressed while others significantly improved my mood. Not all songs by an artist or group had the same effect. However, I had noticed that almost without exception, listening to hard rock or heavy metal music really loudly had consistently had a positive effect on my well-being.

I needed to set up an experiment to see whether or not sound waves could cancel the effects of the fault line's electromagnetic waves, eliminating their ability to cause symptoms in my body.

For the first test I selected a variety of hard rock and heavy metal tunes. The plan was to drive over the fault zones while listening to the songs loudly enough to make an impact yet without impairing my ability to drive safely.

By the time I returned from my expedition, I was exhausted. I had discovered a few new fault zones and although the music had indeed provided some protection against the feelings of despair that often accompanied the other symptoms, I wasn't able to raise my insulation from the physical effects any higher than what the bracelets were providing; in my estimation, sixty percent improvement. I still felt as if someone were squeezing me too tightly and I had difficulty breathing, along with an almost constant need to yawn; yawns that wouldn't complete. Even so, I decided to add the music remedy to my growing arsenal of treatments and continue experimenting.

A few days later I felt an increasing sense of hopelessness. This had become my cue that the symptoms were increasing in severity to a point where an all out panic would not be far behind unless I intervened somehow. It was the perfect opportunity to try out the music therapy. I slipped into my office and put on headphones, experimenting with various tunes until I found a handful that made a positive impact. The experiment was a success. Not only did I keep the panic from taking hold, I had successfully pushed back the feelings of hopelessness.

I organized the tunes into a playlist on my iPod, filing it away for future use. I smiled. I now had another effective weapon in my slowly expanding cache.

My adrenals were under constant stress. Because of the almost constant sensation of being squeezed too tightly my mind would repeatedly hit the panic button, instructing me to run, to get away from the danger.

But run from what? There was no one anywhere near me. I wasn't literally being squeezed; it just felt that way. I would have difficulty breathing, a need to take deep breaths, but for no understandable reason; it wasn't as if I'd just exerted myself through exercise or any physical effort.

My mind's inability to resolve these mixed messages resulted in a frequent state of fight or flight; an appropriate stress response programmed into our DNA. However, this constant flood of chemicals took their toll on my health and my emotions.

I never knew when the symptoms would suddenly worsen, or why, and my body wasn't able to reconcile that the cause of all this hoopla was invisible.

It wasn't a virus or bacterial infection I could fight off. It wasn't an allergy I could take pills for. I couldn't go through a 12-step program and find relief. I didn't entirely understand it and anomalies would crop up constantly, leaving me feeling baffled, if not a little insane.

"You are not crazy," my husband would tell me and I was grateful. I certainly felt as if I was losing it. I was frustrated that even with all my knowledge and experience, I was only able to achieve marginal improvement.

◊ TWELVE ◊

A BREAK IN THE CASE

"WHY did this suddenly get so bad?" I asked days later, my arms thrown up in frustration as I paced the floor of my office. "I know I've had the fatigue and the sleep problems since we moved in here back in 2005, but I never had trouble breathing. Why did that start up in June?"

Aaron had no theories.

"And why did the fatigue suddenly become so incapacitating starting in April 2008?"

I continued pacing and wracked my brain for answers. What had changed? I froze and looked at Aaron.

"I know what it is. I can't believe it but I know what it is; I know what set this thing into overdrive."

In April of 2008, a local telecommunications provider upgraded their infrastructure to accommodate the expanding need for Internet access. I remembered the timing because one of the provider's employees came to our home while we were having other work done. He wanted to test our line. After confirming it was working, he enthusiastically told me about the infrastructure improvements and a new service that would soon be available.

That same month, almost to the day, I began to periodically experience terrible fatigue that was practically debilitating. This is also when, out of the blue, I began to suffer allergy symptoms. From April 2008 until I discovered the bracelets in July 2009, I suffered from a constant runny nose, burning, watery eyes, extreme fatigue and random bouts of hopelessness.

As I continued to discuss the timing in detail with Aaron, more facts came to light.

In December of 2008, the telecommunications provider began offering their new service in our area. Although we elected not to subscribe, within a few weeks, additional, more sinister symptoms began.

In addition to bouts of hopelessness, I had to fight occasional feelings of deep despair, that there was nothing to look forward to in life, that things would never get better, and worst of all, the strong feeling that I was dying.

In the midst of this onslaught I'd launched an all out offensive against the torment. I ate a diet that most would consider healthy, I stepped up my exercise routine, and I tried numerous natural therapies and supplements. Nothing helped. I also spent a number of hours consulting with friends of mine, troubleshooting what was going on.

As I stood in the office that summer day in 2009, a sense of relief came over me. All those months I'd known, deep down, that whatever was happening to me was not psychological, mental, or emotional. I knew I was healthy, even if I felt like I was dying. I knew that whatever was happening was directly related to where I lived and now I had proof.

The new knowledge also provided a possible explanation for the cyclical nature of symptom severity. We lived very close to a strip mall and an office park. If the symptoms intensified as a result of a new technology it would make sense that they would be worse during business hours, when more people would be taking advantage of that new technology.

I was stunned by the revelation but I couldn't argue with the facts. The timing was more than a coincidence; it was a solid lead.

◊ THIRTEEN ◊

RIDING THE WAVES

KNOWING that the infrastructure upgrade had somehow set my system off wasn't enough. I needed to know, specifically, what it was about the new technology that could be causing the problem. It had been a few years since I'd worked in the networking industry but I still had a good grasp of the technology involved, how it had evolved, and had a pretty good understanding of where it was headed.

In the early days of networking, data was transmitted over coaxial cable with an inner conductor surrounded by a tubular insulating layer made from a flexible material which was then surrounded by shielding material made of braided copper strands. The advantage of coaxial cable was that the electromagnetic field carrying the signal existed only in the space between the inner and outer conductors. This allowed the cable to be installed next to metal objects without power loss and provided protection from external electromagnetic interference.

Over time the technology industry evolved and the personal computer revolutionized the way the world did business. As a result, networking needs grew at an exponential rate. The sheer volume of data being transmitted, not to mention the various data types, helped usher in the use of a newer, higher capacity medium; fiber optic cable.

Unlike the electrical signals that were transmitted across a conductive material in coaxial cabling, fiber optic signals were actually light transmitted across bundles of thin strands of glass. These light signals were a different part of the electromagnetic spectrum with a different frequency; one better able to accommodate the ever growing need for increased bandwidth capacity.

Having received government approval to use this different frequency, the technology company upgraded the local infrastructure in April of 2008. Research revealed that the new frequency was the same frequency emitted by the electronic ballasts used with fluorescent lighting. This was significant indeed.

Fluorescent lighting has long been associated with a variety of human health issues, including headaches, eyestrain, fatigue, and even behavioral problems. I remembered a particularly intriguing article I'd read in *San Diego* magazine several years before.

In the mid-80s a Southern California school district built a brand new school that had no windows to allow natural sunlight into the classrooms. Not long after they noticed a variety of health issues, including serious behavioral problems, in their students.

As for myself, I'd experienced problems with fluorescent lighting since I was in second grade. My eyes watered and burned to the point where I was sent to have an eye exam. No issues turned up; my eyesight was fine. Later, when listening to lectures at college, in halls with no windows, I would become so fatigued I almost fell asleep. Given that most classrooms and corporate meeting rooms use this type of lighting in the name of power consumption efficiency, burning watery eyes and extreme fatigue can prove challenging indeed.

In April 2008, the telecommunications infrastructure in our neighborhood was upgraded to accommodate the new frequency and in that exact same month I began to experience constant fatigue that would occasionally become so bad I couldn't function normally. This is also when the constant runny nose and watery burning eyes began. Fatigue and burning, watery eyes were the same symptoms I experienced when around fluorescent lighting.

Until I'd discovered the therapeutic value of the bracelets, the only remedy that brought relief was actually leaving the area. Since wearing the bracelets, which I never took off unless I needed to for an experiment, I no longer had any allergy symptoms and the fatigue wasn't nearly as bad. Best of all, I no longer experienced the periodic three days of debilitating exhaustion.

Although the technology upgrade provided an explanation as to why the symptoms suddenly worsened beginning in April 2008, and even why they appeared to keep business hours, it didn't complete the picture.

Even within those business hours, sometimes the symptom severity would increase dramatically, bringing the corresponding suffering. Additionally, there were other times and other locations where I would also experience a significant increase in symptom intensity. Obviously, I had more work to do.

◊ FOURTEEN ◊

SHAKE, RATTLE AND ROLL

THEY say truth is stranger than fiction and God knows, my life had certainly gone where I'd never been; yet it was about to take another twist. I could predict earthquakes.

On July 21, 2009, I noticed that I felt particularly bad. It was after six pm, the time by when the intensity had usually reduced. However, the level of dizziness and nausea were at an all-time high, and I found the tightness in my chest very uncomfortable. As I stood in our living room talking to Aaron about the intensity of the symptoms, I blurted out, "I bet we're going to have an earthquake tonight, around 3am."

I don't know why I said that. I knew we lived in a target rich environment but the connection between how I felt and the imminence of an earthquake was completely unconscious at this point.

The next morning I woke up feeling fine. The symptoms were almost non-existent. I thought about my prediction and went to check the USGS website. Sure enough, there had been a small earthquake on a nearby fault. I stared at the time; 3:28am. I had been right on.

That I was so close in guessing the exact time had to be a fluke, I thought.

However, I was able to repeat this ability again a few days later when I predicted we would have an earthquake between noon and one in the afternoon on August 2. We had a quake at 12:31pm that was again followed by a significant reduction in symptoms.

I turned it into a game, feeling partly awed and partly horrified by this ability. I laughed uneasily as I envisioned my life becoming a circus sideshow attraction. Still, I continued to try and predict the quakes, wanting to understand the nature of this phenomenon. I even purchased a pocket planner to keep track of the symptoms and predictions[6].

On August 25, I noticed the symptoms had again become quite intense. I talked to Aaron and told him, "I'm going to be sick for three days. We'll have a quake on Friday and then I'll feel better." The next day I told him, "It might be Saturday, but I still think it'll be Friday, around 2pm."

On Friday afternoon, we were sitting at the dining room table.

"I feel better."

We stared at each other in silence for a moment.

"I have to go check."

We had had an earthquake after 1pm. I had again hit the mark. I wasn't surprised when we had another quake on Saturday morning, after which I felt good for the rest of the weekend until, beginning Sunday evening, my symptoms again increased in intensity.

On September 12, I noticed that the symptoms I felt were particularly intense. I was having a great deal of difficulty breathing. I also felt fatigue. By the middle of the 13th, I was feeling horribly fatigued and as if someone had poured molasses on my brain. It was difficult to concentrate.

I hadn't actively tried to predict a quake in a few weeks and figured I had nothing to lose. I decided that on Tuesday morning, early, we would have a quake and I would feel better afterward. I shared this information with Aaron.

On Tuesday morning, as I sat at the computer, I realized I was feeling better. I checked the USGS website. We had had an earthquake at 4am that morning.

I knew I had said early in the morning but I was still surprised it was that early. I had imagined closer to 7am.

As fantastical as it seemed that I was able to predict earthquakes, there was actually a logical explanation. For several years, the USGS, along with scientists from around the world, had been investigating the phenomena of increased EMF emissions from fault lines in the hours and days prior to an earthquake[7].

Since I am affected by these emissions on a daily basis, it made sense that an increase in their output would result in an increase in my symptom severity. This was also consistent with the fact that although my symptoms became significantly worse just prior to an earthquake, once the quake happened, my symptoms reduced back to baseline. The data from studies of the relationship between increased EMFs and earthquakes showed similar findings; the EMF levels reset back to *normal* after the quake.

At this point I had been rating my symptoms on a scale of 1 to 10 and most of the time they hovered between 3 and 5. However, there were occasions when the intensity rose to a 9/10. This was consistently in the hours and days prior to an earthquake on a nearby fault.

I also noticed a relationship between the severity of the symptoms and the number of subsequent quakes as well as their magnitude. Symptoms that were particularly severe were followed by numerous smaller quakes spaced close together, or one larger one.

Although I was consistently able to determine the day and approximate hour of a coming earthquake, I initially avoided trying to predict either magnitude or fault location. Truthfully, I was more interested in finding relief from the extreme discomfort that the symptoms of EMF Sensitivity brought. I considered the ability to predict quakes just another symptom and made no effort to try and develop it. However, as I soon discovered, the body has a mind of its own.

We were driving home from Danville one afternoon when I suddenly experienced a sharp pain in my right ear. It felt as if someone was stabbing me with a letter opener. I instinctively knew that a new symptom had revealed itself. With a sigh, I updated my husband and blurted out that there would be an earthquake in Danville that afternoon, giving him the approximate time and a magnitude of 1.7.

It was really no surprise to learn upon checking the USGS website later that evening, that a magnitude 1.6 earthquake had hit Danville within minutes of my prediction.

Without consciously trying, my body had learned to associate the severity of symptoms with a lead-time prior to an earthquake, as well as the distance from the fault line and magnitude of the event.

◊ FIFTEEN ◊

LOCATION, LOCATION, LOCATION

WHILE all this was transpiring, my family was facing another job-related relocation. In light of what we had learned in July, Aaron and I felt it essential that we make sure wherever we were moving would not present the same difficulties for me.

In reviewing the history of symptoms, locations, and timing, we agreed that geologic fault lines were, by far, the biggest concern. After all, I'd been exposed to the same networking technology away from fault zones and experienced minimal, if any, discomfort.

Unfortunately, the state we were moving to, like so many others in our country, had plenty of fault zones. Before going through with the relocation we had to determine whether or not there was an area we could move to that would be far enough away from them that my health would not be negatively impacted.

So, in August 2009, armed with an AAA TripTik and with more than a little trepidation, we set out on what would be a weeklong road trip.

Since I was playing navigator, I would flip the pages to mark our progress and scope out towns where we were likely to find decent restaurants and lodging for the night. I also took the opportunity to write the locations where I felt EMF symptoms directly onto the TripTik. I noted where the symptoms started and stopped, their severity, and any other details I felt relevant. I made sure to dictate this information to Aaron whenever I drove.

Because I had cell coverage throughout most of the trip I was able to do real-time research into the areas where I felt symptoms. It was no surprise that I was able to consistently identify fault zones in California, Nevada, Utah, Wyoming, and Colorado. In fact, it was a bit of a relief. Whenever there was an absence of symptoms, which was whenever I was away from the fault zones, I felt so good I often found myself wondering if I hadn't imagined it all. Then I would have difficulty breathing or experience severe vertigo and a quick Google search would verify the presence of a fault. This consistency somehow made it all the more real and helped me feel sane.

By the time we returned to California we knew we could go forward with the move. We were relieved to have discovered that there were parts of the country I could live and be free of the terrible symptoms. Even my toddlers were thrilled for me and were excited to move where there were no fault lines.

While the details of the relocation were being worked out I concentrated on the EMF Sensitivity, researching and experimenting. I copied notes from the earthquake journal and my spiral notebook onto my hard drive. I also continued to search for remedies that would alleviate the symptoms.

By far, the greatest relief had come from the metal jewelry. As long as I wore the bracelets, I no longer experienced allergy symptoms or feelings of hopelessness and I felt a nice increase in energy. However, I still struggled with difficulty breathing and a sensation of being squeezed too tightly. I also had episodes of severe vertigo.

One day in September 2009, as I sat at my computer fighting a wave of dizziness, I noticed that the veins on my wrists were once again enlarged and close to the surface. I stared at the phenomenon, pondering the amazing ability of the body to instinctively know when the symptoms were worsening and to respond by drawing more of the beneficial metals through the skin.

By this time I had confirmed the cumulative effect of the metals and wore nine bracelets in addition to the stainless steel band of my watch. And while only getting totally away from fault lines resulted in complete absence of symptoms, I was able to experience between sixty-five and seventy percent improvement with this combination.

Another wave of dizziness washed over me and I struggled to take a breath. I was still staring at the copper bracelets. I wondered; would putting the metals closer to the symptoms bring relief?

At that moment I would have said the worst of the symptoms was the vertigo. I didn't think earrings made of copper, silver, and brass would contain enough of the helpful metals and I felt I would look ridiculous wearing a copper tiara, so I turned my thoughts to respiration. In addition to difficulty taking a breath, I frequently felt as if someone were sitting on my chest and squeezing my solar plexus. Would wearing the metals closer to this area bring an improvement?

A quick search of my jewelry box revealed very little to experiment with. I jumped online and visited a variety of websites, selecting a few inexpensive pieces that were handcrafted from copper, silver, and brass. While I waited for their delivery I wore a small charm made from sterling silver on a stainless steel chain. Not surprisingly, I didn't notice any improvement.

Within two weeks I had a handful of charms on the chain, but in spite of my certainty that I was onto something, I did not notice an improvement in symptoms. I stood before a mirror and studied the necklace in my reflection. Would I need to add additional charms? I worried about this because if the necklace became too heavy I would end up with a stiff and sore neck from all the weight. I continued to stare at the necklace, my eyes going to the chain. It was stainless steel, rather far down the list of insulating metals.

"I need to go shopping," I declared. "I need to go downtown to that silver store, Sterling Works."

I had a brief conversation with the sales clerk and she helped me choose a chain of silver. I transferred all the charms to the new chain and left, eager to see if I felt a difference. Within minutes I was able to breathe more freely and the sensation of being squeezed too tightly became nonexistent.

◊ SIXTEEN ◊

NEW LOCATIONS, NEW SOURCES

ABOUT this time we decided another trip to Colorado was in order. We wanted to narrow down exactly where we would be moving and make initial arrangements for temporary living. I printed a new TripTik and again noted locations where I felt symptoms or their absence.

Since we'd varied the route slightly, I was able to confirm my ability to detect the location of fault lines based on how I was feeling without worrying that I was only remembering the locations from our previous trip. Once again I observed that I felt really good in areas marked by the presence of mining operations. In particular, silver mines. Interestingly, the mines did not have to be active for me to feel the benefits. Even driving through old ghost towns brought not only relief from symptoms, but also a feeling of well-being that included mental clarity and a surge in energy.

Once we'd arrived in Colorado, we focused on the Front Range, which is the residential corridor that runs along I-25. I noted areas where I felt symptoms. Unfortunately, some of the cities I would have loved to move to were also places I had difficulty breathing and a mild vertigo, so I had to cross them off the list. Apparently, there were fault lines in the area.

I was able to eliminate telecommunications technology as a source of concern even though it created a problem for me back in the East Bay. The key was the presence of fault lines. If I was exposed to the same technology away from fault lines, I felt no negative impact.

At one point we found a beautiful area south of Denver where I felt great but I still had to cross it off the list. The surrounding cities were criss-crossed by fault zones. I would have suffered from symptoms, not at home, but every time I went shopping, out to eat, to the library, or any number of other everyday tasks.

On our return trip I continued to validate a match between symptoms felt and the presence of fault lines, as well as the consistent feeling of well being near old mining communities.

"It's too bad we couldn't move to an old ghost town," I murmured as we made our way along I-70 out of Colorado.

Once back in California we focused all our energy on relocation efforts. Thanks to everything I'd learned, by the time we put our house on the market, I had significantly improved my quality of life relative to what it had been only four months before. I continued to experience an increase in the number and severity of symptoms in the hours and days prior to an earthquake, but I also had a sizable arsenal of remedies from which I could draw in order to feel better.

The jewelry remained at the core of my therapies. As long as I wore the bracelets I suffered no allergy symptoms and had an increase in energy. While wearing the necklace with its charms of copper, silver, and brass, the feeling of being squeezed too tightly and the difficulty breathing were almost completely eliminated. And if things got too bad I could spend the day in San Francisco, where there are no fault lines.

By December, we were living in our new state. Because we didn't want to spend Christmas in a hotel, we paid a visit to family in the Midwest. Interestingly, while driving back, we hit a stretch of highway where I began to feel sick.

"If I didn't know any better I'd think there were fault lines near here," I said to Aaron. "I feel like someone poured molasses on my brain."

Whipping out my cell phone I plugged in the search criteria.

"I don't believe it. I mean, I should, I guess. We're driving near the New Madrid fault zone[8]." I looked over at Aaron. "Well, at least it's consistent."

Until that point I had never heard of the New Madrid fault zone. I did not associate the Midwest with large fault zones, though I had experienced the occasional earthquake while growing up there.

In early January we moved into our new home and although I felt really good I wanted to learn more. For instance, I was interested in discovering more remedies. Fortunately, I had an inverse situation from what I had been dealing with in California. I now lived in an area with a lower than national average of seismic activity. However, I lived within easy driving distance to plenty of research material.

For instance, on previous visits I had observed that I consistently experienced certain symptoms while near the Denver Tech Center. I felt as if I was being squeezed too tightly and I had difficulty breathing. This jarred a memory for me.

While with a previous employer I had traveled regularly to Colorado, including annual training conferences at the Denver Tech Center. I remembered that the last time I had been there for training I experienced an episode of difficulty breathing. Because I noticed this right after lunch, someone suggested I may be having some sort of allergic reaction to something I ate and suggested I try Benadryl[©]. The gift shop carried the allergy medication and sure enough, I felt relief within a short time of taking it.

In light of the current situation I wondered if perhaps all those years ago I had been feeling the effects of fault lines. Colorado certainly has its share of them[9]. Attributing the symptoms to fault lines rather than a food allergy was not as relevant as the fact that the Benadryl had made a difference. I wondered if that would still be true.

The city of Boulder is beautiful, and we definitely would have given it serious consideration as a hometown, but for one little detail. The EMF symptoms were extremely strong there.

One day in February 2010, I hopped in the car with my family and a Benadryl tablet. Because I knew this medication caused sleepiness I took up position as a passenger while Aaron drove. We knew exactly where in Boulder the symptoms started from previous visits. Shortly before arriving, I took one of the allergy tablets so it had time to kick in during our visit. I'd made a point of not wearing the bracelets or necklace so I could determine the extent, if any, of the benefits of the allergy medication.

At the exact location I'd felt the symptoms previously, they started up. I had trouble breathing, felt as if I were being squeezed too tightly and had that annoying, continuous yawning that wouldn't complete. I also felt phlegm in my throat and my eyes began to water and burn. I instructed Aaron to follow the identical route we had traveled on our most recent trip, including a couple of wrong turns we'd made. Within about ten minutes the Benadryl was in my system and I was pleased to note that it had a beneficial effect. The symptoms reduced significantly; about a ninety percent improvement. I had successfully found a new addition for my cache of remedies. Pleased with the results of my most recent experiment, we returned home, an area free from EMF influence.

Or so I thought.

◊ SEVENTEEN ◊

TECHNOLOGY PLAYS A ROLE

ONE afternoon in early February 2010, I noticed I was feeling extremely fatigued. In fact, for two days in a row I had taken a nap, which would be a shock to anyone who knows me. I'm not and never have been a successful napper. In fact, I typically feel so much worse after a nap that I go to great lengths to avoid them.

Given everything we'd been through in the last months, not to mention we'd only been in our new home for about five weeks, many people might suggest it was simply the stress, both physical and mental, of relocating to a new area, in the snowy winter no less. However, I knew it wasn't.

For one thing, other than suffering the symptoms from the EMF Sensitivity, I was pretty healthy. Instead of the typical respiratory infection most of us get every one to two years, I had only been sick twice in the previous ten. I maintained a relatively healthy lifestyle, exercising regularly and eating pretty well. I regularly practiced stress reduction techniques, including meditation. I had not suffered from post-partum depression and was consistently able to handle the stresses of life. I had felt so good since moving, in fact, that over the months of January and February I had weaned myself of the protective jewelry. Since we lived in an area free from geologic fault lines, I felt no need for them.

After waking up from the second nap I discussed the sudden onset of fatigue with Aaron. He began careful questioning about when it started and what may have changed in that timeframe. Thankfully, he was still quick to consider technology as a culprit, even as I focused most of my theories on fault line emissions.

"It started Tuesday?" he said. "That's when I hooked up the DVD player so the kids could watch a movie."

At that point we were still unpacking and not all our home electronics were set up.

"You know, I never used to go in the family room back in California," I pointed out, "and that's where the DVD player was."

"Why don't we unplug the DVD player to test it out?" he suggested.

Within minutes of doing so I felt much better.

Further discussion brought to light that at the same time he had hooked up my laser printer.

"Let's unplug that as well," he advised.

I felt even better once we did, so of course I wanted to know what it was about those two devices that could be causing the problem. First, I had to consider what they had in common. Aaron pointed out that they both used lasers, so that is where I started my research. Since I was dealing with electromagnetic frequencies, I turned first to understanding how the lasers were powered.

In North America, electricity supplied by the power company is Alternating Current (AC) in which the direction of the current's flow is reversed or alternated 110 to 120 times per second. Most electronic devices, including DVD players and laser printers, require Direct Current (DC) in which the current flows in the same direction at all times. In order for these devices to be powered then, the AC needs to be converted to DC. A device known as a rectifier or converter does this. This conversion can be done within the device itself or externally, such as the power brick used in laptop power cords.

Previous research into fluorescent lighting had revealed that because of the fluctuations inherent in the nature of alternating current, there were quick, repeated changes in light intensity; light that appeared to flutter and be unsteady. This is known as flicker. The type of ballast, which controls the electrical supply to fluorescent lights, affects the amount of flicker.

It is suspected that for the percentage of the population who are able to perceive this flicker, negative health symptoms occur, including headaches and migraines, eyestrain, and general discomfort[10]. Personally, I can add extreme fatigue and mental confusion to that list, two symptoms I have to fight every time I'm in a grocery store and most retail stores.

Supposedly, the problem has been addressed in newer compact fluorescent bulbs because the electronic ballasts take the current and convert it to voltages at a much higher frequency. The result is a flicker frequency that is apparently so high that the human eye cannot detect any fluctuations in the light intensity. I have to admit, we use these newer bulbs in our home and I have not experienced any negative symptoms from them.

In thinking of the DVD player and considering the nature of alternating current I wondered if the same fluctuations might be resulting in some sort of electromagnetic noise that leaked from the converter itself. Even though I wouldn't be able to perceive such a fluctuation visually, I couldn't rule it out nor the idea that it was having a negative effect; in particular, extreme fatigue.

I discussed my suspicions with both Aaron and Derek, the engineer who had suggested the blind driving test in California. Derek pointed out that in most cases there would be a filtration circuit that minimizes the ripple or AC leakage current from the converter. He said that in some cases the current might run through a DC-to-DC converter as the DC voltage needs are different for the various electronic components that make up the product. He added that there is always a ripple in the DC side of the circuit of these devices, adding that in high end audio equipment, the manufacturers go to great expense to filter as much out as possible, coming up with all kinds of innovative ways of doing it. For common devices, however, he suggested manufacturers likely do the minimum, just enough that the devices function.

Aaron added that the DVD player we had wasn't of the highest quality and pointed out that it was older.

"Either way," he advised, "we should buy a new one."

I told him I was happy to replace it with a newer model but I wanted to have the final say on our selection. I believed that I would be able to feel a problem even in a retail store that was filled with electronics and was likely to use fluorescent lighting. Our next stop? Best Buy electronics store.

I had a brief conversation with the sales associate and he helped us select a model to try. He plugged the model in and I immediately felt some sort of electromagnetic effect. I reached my hand out and was surprised to find that the model, manufactured by a reputable company I associated with high quality products, actually vibrated, as if there was some sort of mechanical defect. Aaron noticed the vibration and said we needed to try another model.

The associate selected another brand and plugged the device in, being sure to insert a DVD so that the laser itself was engaged. I had no problem with the second model and we went ahead with the purchase. I reflected on the irony that the brand was one I had never heard of.

In an effort to find a good answer I focused my research on how the laser printer and DVD player utilized power. I consulted a friend who is an electrical engineer. Interestingly, Brook didn't conclude that it was the converter for the laser. He explained that most motors in small devices are DC and confirmed that there is electrical interference with these motors. The question was how much they gave off and how close a person was to them. He suggested that since I am a receptor for a lot of EMF noises I would pick up on the interference long before anyone else. Derek and Aaron agreed with his assessment.

Several weeks went by and I was happy to note that I had no problems with the new DVD player. Unfortunately, I could not say the same about the laser printer. Even when the printer was not in use, as long as it was plugged in I felt symptoms. I realized the same thing had been true of the old DVD player. Even when a movie wasn't playing I suffered terrible fatigue, only getting relief when it was unplugged. Even though I couldn't pinpoint the exact cause, it was clear to me that something about the electrical nature of these products was giving me grief.

Brook had pointed out, as Aaron and Derek had, that the FCC[11], which regulates interstate and international communications by radio, television, wire, satellite and cable in the US, sets standards by which manufacturers must comply. These include safety standards.

Additionally, I knew from my years in technology that the Institute of Electronics Engineers (IEEE)[12] developed standards involved with their charter of advancing technology related to electricity. These standards also address issues of safety.

However, I argued that standards were simply guidelines unless laws and regulations made compliance with them compulsory. Additionally, the parameters of safety addressed by these standards generally apply to the average citizen. When it comes to EMF Sensitivity, current research suggests that only between 1.5 and 3 percent of the population suffers from EMF Sensitivity,[13] and while I personally suspect the number is higher, we are still talking about a small percentage of the population overall. It is not practical to expect a complete overhaul of decades of work for a small percentage of the population.

In fact, it was in great part because of this reality, not to mention my own personal experiences, that I set out to discover ways to reduce and/or eliminate the symptoms from EMF Sensitivity.

I have never had any issues with the DVD drives in laptops or desktop computers, or with any number of electronic appliances, including a TiVo box, satellite converter box, CD players, or a variety of other home appliances.

Derek advised me that the laser transport motors in a CD player are far less complex than in a DVD player and probably emit a much different frequency and transient characteristics than CD players.

In the end I decided that since I was quite happy with the laser printer, I was more than willing to simply unplug it when it was not in use. After all, for the short duration I have it plugged in, I do not suffer enough to justify replacing the model.

◊ EIGHTEEN ◊

THE INNER LIMITS

IN late March 2010, I began suffering from an intense headache and jaw pain similar to TMJ. Because we were starting the spring season when thunderstorms and atmospheric changes were common I initially suspected the cause was EMFs from the erratic weather that, in our location, seemed to change every six to eighteen hours.

About this same time I began having difficulty sleeping. I was waking up approximately every sixty to ninety minutes throughout the night and had a great deal of difficulty falling back to sleep. This continued every night.

After two weeks the weather improved but I still had difficulty sleeping and the pain in my head and jaw continued. As a result I began to search for other causes.

I drove around to see if a change in location made a difference. It was negligible, so I considered the home. I was puzzled because I figured I would have noticed a problem when we'd first moved in, not four months later. Considering further, I realized that I felt worse when in two rooms in our home; my office and my bedroom. What made that significant was that the office is directly above the other room.

We had been out that day to see if a change in location made a difference in my symptoms. It didn't. When we got back I suggested we unplug every electrical device in my office, including two small lamps, to see if I felt a difference in the bedroom. Surprisingly, I did. In fact, I slept very well that night. Obviously, something in my office was causing a problem. What interested me was the idea that EMFs were apparently forming an invisible vertical wall, affecting me not only while I was in my office, but also whenever I was in the room directly below it.

Aaron and I came up with a plan. The next morning he would go up to my office and try plugging and unplugging various electronics to see if it made a difference. Because I have always been able to hear the electrical hum associated with alarm systems, computers, and home appliances, I told him I would enter the bedroom first to see if I noticed a difference in there. I didn't want the sound (or lack of) from the appliances to influence my observations in the office.

By the time we were through we knew what the problem was and had figured out a very simple solution.

"I wish I'd had a camera," Aaron said. "You nailed it every time."

To explain the problem in full context I need to go back to the FCC and IEEE. These organizations are responsible for the safety specifications of, among other things, technology related to electricity. Part of the process involves some pretty rigorous testing after which they release their findings to various organizations, all accompanied by the appropriate documentation. The information released includes the maximum threshold of the devices and circuits that have been tested.

We discovered that the sheer number of electronic devices located in my office created EMF difficulties for two reasons.

First, some of them, including a couple of audio speakers I had plugged into my computer, required a lot of electricity. For each device we added we increased the likelihood of power leakage due to the electrical system approaching its maximum specification.

Secondly, we had several of the appliances plugged into one power strip. The power cords were literally touching as every port on the strip was filled. It became obvious to Aaron after some trial and error that there was electrical interference between the cords as a result.

The solution was two-fold. First, we discussed which appliances could be relocated to another part of the house. I told him I didn't need the external speakers. Additionally, one of the printers was wireless so it could be located anywhere in the house. Everything that didn't need to be there was moved.

The second part of the solution involved reallocating the way the remaining electronics in my office were plugged in.

The results were immediate. I felt a huge improvement and within twelve hours the pain in my head was gone. Within forty-eight hours the pain in my jaw had disappeared. Beginning the first night I'd unplugged all the electronics and continuing after we relocated and redistributed the devices, my sleep improved.

Once I was no longer in pain I could focus on some interesting observations made during the testing.

The EMFs had formed an invisible vertical wall that went from the office straight down into my bedroom. It was located in the exact same place in both rooms, approximately three feet past the doorway. If I took three steps into either room I felt the unpleasant sensations.

I also noticed something peculiar; something I suspected was significant. I could hear and feel the EMFs as a heavy silence.

If anyone has ever tried out a pair of noise canceling headphones[14], they have experienced the silence that comes once the headphones are turned on. What they are actually *hearing* is the noise canceling frequency. The waves entering the ear cause the brain to register silence.

"Imagine that same feeling of silence all over your body," I told Aaron.

It was the most accurate description I could give. In addition to painful and uncomfortable sensations, I *heard* a silence that actually penetrated my entire body; presenting itself as an invisible wall. It was like a heaviness; a heavy silence. When the offending appliances were unplugged, the rooms felt clear and sound was experienced normally.

In late June I gained additional insight into this phenomenon. I was editing the manuscript when I realized I felt incredibly fatigued and as if someone had poured molasses on my brain. When I found myself rereading the same sentence but still not comprehending it I knew something was wrong; something EMF-related. I looked around the space where I was working in our dining room. Aaron's laptop was less than two feet away but I knew that wasn't the problem. We often worked in close proximity and I never recalled it being a problem. I glanced around. There was a home entertainment appliance sitting on the floor. That was new.

The device was one of two we used to stream music wirelessly. Because Aaron had been using it for something else entirely, nothing was hooked up to it. The device just sat on the floor plugged into the wall. I unplugged it and the symptoms disappeared. I plugged it back in and they came back within seconds. I told Aaron what was going on and we began the all-too-common analysis of what might be going on in the world of EMFs.

What immediately came to light was the fact that the other wireless streaming device, located in another room, did not cause a problem for me. So, what was the difference between the two? The one in our dining room had an amp in it and the other one did not. Aaron then pointed out that the large speaker in my office had also had an amp in it. He brought the non-amp streaming device into the dining room and plugged it in. I had no problems. He checked the power draw on each and pointed out that there was a significantly higher draw on the one with the amp in it.

I consulted Derek because, as an audiophile, he is able to provide a unique perspective of audio equipment and its components. He theorized that WiFi in the presence of an amp device was causing a problem for me. He suggested that we shut off all the wireless devices in our home and then plug the amp devices in and see what happens.

When the WiFi alone is plugged in I have no difficulty. It's a dual-band B-G access point. When the amp devices alone are plugged in they do not cause any problems for me. However, when the amp devices are plugged in while the WiFi is going I experience symptoms that vary depending on the device and how close I am to it.

The large powered speaker is the worst. I feel a burning electrical sensation in my lower spine and flowing down my right leg. I also have mucous in the back of my throat.

The streaming device is next. It feels as if someone has poured molasses on my brain and I have difficulty concentrating. I feel very tired and lethargic. I also had burning watery eyes. While this may seem worse than the symptoms related to the speakers, it isn't. When Aaron turned on the speakers, the electrical sensation that flowed down my leg was so painful I leapt from my chair and yelled at him to turn it off.

In the living room, the powered speakers, which are a different make and model from the one I had in my office, presented the least difficulty. I got a headache on my left side that disappeared the moment the WiFi was turned off. However, the longer I sat near them when the access device was on, the more symptoms I got and the worse they became. I had difficulty breathing and had that annoying yawning that wouldn't complete.

By the time the experiment was over I was exhausted. I felt as if I'd been beat up. I also felt as if my nerves were quite raw and my body had been placed on "red alert." I felt a residual effect that spiked about five minutes after the testing was done. In order to help *reset* my system, I put on headphones and played songs from my remedy list at high volume. After just one song I felt better.

So, what was happening?

I believe that we all have a threshold of tolerance when it comes to the various electromagnetic frequencies. When this limit has been surpassed, we can experience symptoms of EMF Sensitivity. I think that the amp within an electrical device actually amplifies the WiFi frequency to a level that is beyond my tolerance. As a result, when I am in the presence of this combination, I experience symptoms.

◊ NINETEEN ◊

LIFE AS A CONTINUING EXPERIMENT

DETERMINED not to let EMF Sensitivity rule my life, I worked to discover as many therapies as possible. Even though I lived in an area that had no fault lines, simply driving around often resulted in symptoms since there are fault zones scattered throughout the state, if not the country. Additionally, the spring weather pattern in this part of the country, complete with numerous thunderstorms, frequently brought EMF related symptoms. As a result I have had daily opportunities to learn additional information and discover new remedies.

For instance, one evening we decided to attend a book signing south of Denver. I knew that the drive would take me through stretches of I-25 where I would experience unpleasant symptoms. In fact, the city where the bookstore was located was generally problematic for me.

I kept a packet of Benadryl in the car since it increased relief from the seventy to eighty percent I achieved wearing the jewelry to about ninety percent. However, I wasn't happy with the sleepiness, so I decided to forgo the extra relief in favor of additional energy.

Not long after we left our home I was inspired to pop some chewing gum in my mouth. I also pulled out my cell phone and began to read the news to Aaron. Several articles later I suddenly stopped and took stock.

"I'm not feeling any symptoms," I said in awe. "This is normally where I start to feel bad and I feel fine. It's the gum."

I wasn't certain why, I just knew it was. I pulled the piece out and I immediately began to feel negative symptoms that included the annoying yawning and mucous drainage. I popped the gum back in and within seconds of chewing it the symptoms disappeared.

"You know? I used to chew gum constantly in California, remember?"

In fact I was never without a pack of the stuff in the car as well as two or three in the house.

"I wonder if subconsciously I knew it would help?"

I thought about why the gum was having a positive effect.

"I think it has to do with the way the ear processes sound waves."

I reminded Aaron that I *heard* electricity as a constant low-level hum. I could also hear alarm systems and many computer systems as a low ringing. Interestingly, these tones were accompanied by a feeling of pressure in the area of the ear.

I thought about my recent observation with the vertical EMF wall. I had heard the EMFs as silence and felt them as a sensation of pressure.

"Chewing gum helps pressurize the fluid in the ear canal, which is why it's helpful during take-off and landing. This has to be related somehow."

My mind was off and running. Was it sound or pressure? I needed to test both angles.

"I'll need to try some of those ear plugs you can get at the drugstore. They're for the discomfort felt during elevation changes when flying. I also need to try the Bose headphones. If the noise canceling sound blocks the problematic waves like the heavy metal music does, then not only do I have another remedy, I have an anatomical link."

The next day I tested the earplugs. They had no effect on the symptoms. I then tested the noise canceling headphones and experienced relief, just as I had with the chewing gum. I noticed that the relief came more quickly with chewing gum than with the headphones. Unfortunately, the chewing gum is a bit temporary. Relief only exists while actually chewing the gum and by the end of the experiment, my jaw was tired.

Several days later I was able to make an additional observation regarding symptoms and one of the new remedies. As I sat in my office editing this manuscript, I noticed that the sky outside was rather overcast. A thunderstorm system was coming through. I knew from previous experience that I suffered a variety of health issues when a storm system was approaching, including migraines. I understood from research that it was a result of the EMFs in the atmosphere prior to and during such weather systems.

I had been able to alleviate most of the symptoms simply by wearing the necklace with the copper, silver, and brass charms, in addition to the bracelets. However, the jewelry was unable to prevent the mild feeling of despair that I inevitably experienced when a storm system was present. Fortunately, the level of despair that resulted from the storm system EMFs wasn't nearly as bad as from the fault lines EMFs.

Still, I was not happy to experience any downturn in my mood.

Normally, I would listen to the songs that helped push back those feelings and stabilize my mood. Since removing the speakers from my office I had been using Bose headphones with the iPod to accomplish this. As I was about to turn on the music I paused. I wondered if simply turning on the noise canceling would help.

Sure enough, within a few minutes of activating the headphones, the symptom of despair reduced, eventually disappearing altogether.

I wanted to test the extent to which these two new remedies relieved symptoms. I set up a trip to the grocery store. I always experienced severe fatigue and difficulty concentrating within a short time of entering any retail establishment that used fluorescent lighting.

First I tested the noise canceling headphones. It took a little over a minute but the symptoms disappeared. I turned off the headphones and within a few minutes the symptoms returned. I tried the chewing gum and within seconds the symptoms were gone.

Between the two remedies, chewing gum definitely worked more quickly. However, once I quit chewing the gum, the symptoms returned. When I turned off the noise canceling headphones, I still had a measure of freedom from symptoms. The longer I wore the headphones, the longer I would be symptom free even after turning them off, suggesting a sort of temporary tolerance build-up. I remembered a similar benefit in California. If I spent a few hours away from the fault zones then I would have several hours without symptoms upon returning.

I was certain that there was a link between the way the inner ear processed sound and EMF Sensitivity. The human ear has three main parts, the outer ear, the middle ear, and the inner ear. When sound waves enter the ear and strike the eardrum, it vibrates. The vibrations are passed to the small bones of the middle ear and then transmitted to the inner ear where they become nerve impulses. The brain interprets these impulses as sound.

Most humans hear sound waves with a frequency between 12 Hz and 20 kHz. Problematic EMFs tend to fall outside this range, either higher or lower.

Well, there is a saying: Garbage In/Garbage Out. I believe people who have EMF Sensitivity are actually hearing the EMFs and something about the way the noise is interpreted triggers an immune system response which translates into a host of physical symptoms.

Some people may wonder how anyone could detect frequencies outside the range of sound. To answer that we have to consider what's average. The range assigned to sound waves simply explains what the average human ear is able to hear. Just as with most things in life, there are exceptions.

How was Beethoven able to create such beautiful music if he was deaf? In the book *Think and Grow Rich,* we learn the story of Napoleon Hill's son, who was born without ears and yet learned to hear.

At least three of the individuals I know who are EMF Sensitive have been medically tested and can hear outside the threshold of sound.

EMFs from fault lines are ultra low in frequency; quite a bit lower than 12 Hz. However, many people, including me, claim to hear them; we hear earthquakes before they hit. Theoretically, this shouldn't be possible. However, recent research has demonstrated that it is.[15]

Although more research needs to be done, I think I'm onto something.

PART II

EMF Sensitivity

◊ TWENTY ◊

LIFE'S GOT RHYTHM

FROM ultra-low frequencies produced by the earth's fault lines to high-end cosmic radiation, EMFs are a part of our ecology. It is common knowledge that electromagnetic frequencies at certain parts of the spectrum are dangerous to humans. Great care is taken to protect the public from exposure to these frequencies.

Government and independent agencies do extensive testing aimed at determining safety limits and setting standards based on those limits. The idea that some individuals fall outside the parameters set is not such a far-fetched notion.

Take air bags for instance. The design and deployment of this safety device is modeled after the average citizen. So, where does that leave those who aren't average; who are taller, shorter, lighter, or heavier? My grandmother had to have the airbag in her car disabled; she was only 4' 10."

The same concept of safety testing and guidelines is used when defining the parameters for exposure to and utilization of electromagnetic energies in products and services. Testing is modeled after the average citizen. If we consider the airbag analogy then we can see that sensitivity in some people is not inconceivable.

This is not the stuff of science fiction and certainly nothing new. Nor does sensitivity always translate into discomfort. Someone able to hear beyond the threshold of human hearing is simply someone who is able to audibly detect frequencies higher or lower than most humans. People who see auras are simply able to see a part of the visual spectrum not available to everyone.

However, that being said, I am aware of the debate regarding whether or not certain energy frequencies, particularly those emitted by technology, have an adverse affect on human health. Parties on both sides of this controversial issue feel passionately about their claims and obviously the implications are far reaching with financial repercussions.

Unfortunately, such a debate has acted as a beacon to conspiracy theorists as well as those who love to vilify governments and corporations. As a result, serious research has been compromised; research that could help those who are adversely affected.

By sharing my own story, I hope to reach out to others who are affected, to help them understand that they are not alone, and more importantly, they are not crazy. EMF Sensitivity is real, it's complex, and it is very much misunderstood, even by those who have it.

In the pages that follow I will share theories and research that I believe will provide insight into what EMF Sensitivity is and isn't, and I will suggest various remedies that may offer some relief. Since it is my understanding that there is no cure for this condition, the suggestions are simply tools that may enable those who are EMF sensitive to live a more comfortable life.

My intention in bringing this information to light is not to point fingers or start a crusade. We live in an amazing time where technology improves the quality of millions of lives far beyond simple conveniences. No crystal ball is needed to know that as we evolve, technology will do so right alongside of us. Therefore, my philosophy is that it is far better to exist in harmony with it to the extent that we can.

◊ TWENTY ONE ◊

So, What is EMF Sensitivity?

What is EMF Sensitivity?

In order to adequately answer that question, it's probably best to start out by stating what EMF Sensitivity *isn't*. It isn't a disease. It isn't a virus. It isn't a bacterial infection. It isn't a mental illness. Simply put, it's *a sensitivity*, or an intolerance resulting from exposure to certain electromagnetic frequencies.

Different people are affected by different frequencies and manifest symptoms in different ways. An individual can be affected by multiple frequencies at different levels of the spectrum and each of the different frequencies can cause different symptoms.

Even more confusing are the symptoms themselves. They are symptoms that could indicate any number of conditions and causes, which makes identifying EMF Sensitivity a lengthy and potentially dangerous effort.

In my own situation, it took several years and numerous failed therapies before I was able to identify the true cause of my symptoms and find remedies that worked.

WHAT CAUSES EMF SENSITIVITY?

Why are some people allergic to strawberries or flowers? Why do some people get headaches from red wine? Why do some people get two colds a year while others never report a sick day in their life? Obviously, the answer is far from simple and a variety of factors likely play a role. The truth is, some people are EMF sensitive and some people aren't. It doesn't do any good to try to assign blame because there is none.

However, that being said, I have noticed a relationship between the way the ear processes sound and EMF Sensitivity. I have observed that most individuals who are EMF Sensitive are able to hear beyond audio threshold limits (12 Hz and 20kHz)[16]. We actually hear electromagnetic frequencies, even the ultra low frequencies that precede an earthquake[17].

WHAT IS HAPPENING TO ME?

The human brain, the center of the human nervous system, is an electrochemical organ. Billions of neurons pass signals to each other via trillions of synaptic connections. The brain interprets these signals and issues instructions based on their input. For example, if a nerve impulse signals the brain that the hand is in pain, the brain sends out instructions to not only determine the cause of the pain, but what to do to eliminate it.

In the case of EMF Sensitivity, the problematic frequencies are translated into nerve impulses that the brain interprets as a threat. This elicits an immune response that includes the release of histamine; a compound that increases the permeability to white blood cells in order to allow them to engage foreign invaders in the infected tissues.[18] Histamine also triggers the inflammatory response; the initial response of the body to harmful stimuli.[19] This inflammation results in a number of unpleasant symptoms that can include burning, watery eyes and excess mucous.

Is EMF Sensitivity an allergy?

EMF Sensitivity is similar to an allergy in that the body's immune system is triggered, resulting in a number of unpleasant symptoms, such as burning and watery eyes, fatigue, and a runny nose. However, unlike an allergy, one cannot be exposed to small bits of a trigger and build up tolerance. Additionally, evidence suggests that the longer the exposure to the EMF Sensitivity triggers, the more intolerant the individual becomes.

BRAIN WAVES AND FREQUENCIES

The brain is estimated to generate enough electricity to power a light bulb[20]. This electrical activity is displayed in the form of brainwaves and can be measured by an electroencephalogram. These waves are classified from most active to least active; beta, alpha, theta, and delta.

Beta waves range between 15 and 40 cycles a second and are associated with a mind that is actively engaged, such as when having a conversation.

Alpha waves range between 9 and 14 cycles per second. These are the waves associated with meditation and relaxation.

Theta waves range between 5 and 8 cycles per second. These waves are associated with daydreaming. Many people report an increase in creativity while functioning at this level.

Delta waves range between 1.5 and 4 cycles per second. These waves are associated with a deep sleep that is dreamless.

Research has demonstrated that we cycle through these various states throughout a 24-hour period as a part of normal brain function. Further, even as one brainwave state may dominate, depending on the activity level of the brain, there is a mix of the other three brainwave states at all times.

These waves are like instruments near a tuning fork; they will synchronize to whatever frequency they are exposed to. This is known as entrainment[21]. An example of this would be the use of the alpha centering sound, developed by Jose Silva, to induce deep levels of relaxation[22].

A clear example of brain wave function being negatively impacted by electromagnetic frequencies would be photosensitive epilepsy. Lights flashing between 5 and 30 times per second have been known to induce seizures in some individuals.

Another example of brain wave function being negatively impacted took place in Japan in December 1997. Japanese officials reported that 700 people, primarily school children, were rushed to the hospital after watching a *Pokemon* episode. These individuals suffered convulsions, vomiting, irritated eyes, and other symptoms after a scene in which there was five seconds of flashing red light in the eyes of one of the show's most popular characters; *Pikachu*. When excerpts from the episode were later aired during a TV news show, more children were affected[23].

Michael Persinger, a cognitive neuroscience researcher and university professor, is famous for his use of weak magnetic fields to stimulate people's temporal lobes[24]. He believed that inducing excessive electrical bursts of electricity in the brain would result in subjects having a spiritual experience. He claims that 80% of those tested felt an unexplained presence in the room.

As we can see from these examples, our brain waves are vulnerable. Problems arise when an individual who is EMF Sensitive is exposed to electromagnetic frequencies that are incompatible with the brain's natural rhythm. These rogue frequencies hijack the brain waves, putting them out of normal range.

Compromised brain waves mean compromised instructions transmitted to the body and since the brain is responsible for our survival and well-being, the result is that every function, whether physical, mental, or emotional, can be adversely affected.

WHAT ARE THE SYMPTOMS OF EMF SENSITIVITY?

There are numerous symptoms and different frequencies may elicit different ones. Additionally, the strength of the frequency as well as its proximity can alter the degree to which the symptoms are experienced. Symptoms include:

- Skin irritations, including tingling, burning, and pins and needles sensations
- An unpleasant feeling of warmth/burning sensation to the head similar to a sunburn or fever
- Pressure/heaviness in the head
- Heart rate changes such as tachycardia and arrhythmia
- High blood pressure
- Headaches and tooth aches
- Profound malaise
- Visual changes including blurred vision, watery and burning eyes
- Nausea

- Tinnitus
- Varying degrees of fatigue including exhaustion
- Loss of concentration and memory
- Neurological, respiratory, and gastric problems
- Alteration of sleep pattern and appetite
- Mood swings and depression
- In extreme cases, convulsions and loss of consciousness

Unfortunately, these symptoms can indicate a number of other conditions; so identifying EMF Sensitivity can take a bit of detective work.

How do I know if I have EMF Sensitivity?

EMF Sensitivity can be difficult to identify because it is natural to attribute many of the symptoms to other causes, such as stress or allergies. However, with a bit of sleuthing and a lot of patience, one should be able to figure it out. It would definitely be worth the effort given that taking medications for one malady when it's really another can have dangerous consequences; particularly when medications and lifestyle changes associated with certain therapies are involved.

A journal is an invaluable tool for determining whether or not someone is suffering from EMF Sensitivity. Keeping track of symptoms, severity, and relevant details provides important insight. Pertinent information would include the location where symptoms were felt and whether or not the symptoms went away when away from a certain location. Other helpful facts include the time of day, the season, what activity they were engaged in, anything they had to eat or drink, how much sleep one had and any changes in regular activities. Keep in mind that each individual is unique and may be sensitive to different frequencies and even multiple frequencies at different parts of the spectrum. Additionally, different frequencies may cause different symptoms or alter the severity.

It would be interesting to note the onset of the symptoms and see if anything significant happened at that time. In my own case, I was always sensitive to the ultra low frequencies emitted by fault lines, but after the technology infrastructure in our neighborhood was upgraded, not only was the severity of the symptoms amplified, new ones appeared.

◊ TWENTY TWO ◊

EMF TRIGGERS

WHAT ARE TRIGGERS FOR EMF SENSITIVITY?

Although it is not an allergy, it is handy to use similar terminology when explaining the condition and its causes. There are actually quite a number of potential triggers and not all of them are technological in origin.

THUNDERSTORMS

Many individuals on our planet suffer from migraines and body aches whenever a thunderstorm is imminent. The extremely low frequencies associated with thunderstorms occur between the surface of the earth and its ionosphere, caused when lightning strikes make electrons in the atmosphere oscillate. The range of these frequencies is 200 – 500 Hz.

Fault Lines

In 1980, the Soviets and Japanese began a study of electromagnetic emissions related to earthquakes. In 1991, the Stanford News Service released an article detailing a similar study. Scientists monitoring extremely low frequency (ULF) and very low frequency (VLF) radio waves consistently observed an increase in emissions prior to earthquakes. The range for extremely low frequencies (ELFs) is 1 – 300 Hz and the range for very low frequencies (VLFs) is 3 – 30 kHz.

Volcanoes

In November of 1986, researchers at the Ohshima Volcano Observatory of Tokyo University, east of Motomachi, noted several clear burst-like VLF emissions prior to a volcanic eruption[25]. The same phenomenon was observed again in July of 1989 and has been consistently observed since.

Outer Space

Background radiation in space is composed of high-energy X-rays, gamma rays, and cosmic rays that can all play havoc with the cells in our body. In addition, the sun produces a range of wavelengths from long-wave infrared to short-wavelength ultraviolet (UV) frequencies.

In 2007, NASA and the Canadian Space Agency launched multiple satellites into orbit to study electromagnetic storms in space to gain a better understanding of how they affect the inhabitants of our planet[26]. When these storms reach the earth they affect more than human physiology; they can take out satellites and other technological instruments on the surface[27].

RADIO

Electromagnetic waves with a range between 3 Hz – 300 GHz are called radio waves. Not just emitted by radio stations, radio waves are emitted by stars and gases in space.

SOUND

Sound energy is an oscillation of pressure transmitted through a solid, liquid, or gas, within the range of approximately 12 Hz to 20 kHz, at a level strong enough to be heard by most humans. Sound energy is quite powerful. Depending on the frequency, its vibrations can be either healing or destructive. A glass that shatters after being exposed to operatic voice loud enough and long enough is one example of the destructive power of sound waves. Seismic waves, the sounds radiating from an earthquake, can induce aftershocks that can easily be as destructive, if not more so, than the quake itself. Scientists at Los Alamos have been able to reproduce this phenomenon in the laboratory[28].

The healing properties of music have long been understood. Singing bowls, also known as medicine bowls, have been around for centuries. They can produce a complex chord of harmonic overtones and are typically used to induce a state of meditation and well-being.

In 1839, Heinrich Wilhelm Dove discovered that playing slightly different frequencies separately to each ear produced a perception of interference beats at the same rate as would if physically created. Known as binaural beats or binaural tones, they can be used to synchronize brain waves in order to reduce anxiety and achieve health benefits.

While there has been a strong emphasis on the healing properties of music, perhaps too little attention has been paid to the damaging aspects. It is well understood that listening to music at extremely high volume for extended periods of time will cause nerve damage resulting in hearing loss. However, there are other dangers associated with the frequencies of music. The heart, another electrical organ, can go into arrhythmia when exposed to certain musical beats.

In *Messages from Water*, Dr. Masaru Emoto provides stunning photos that illustrate pattern changes in water molecules after exposure to a variety of sound energies.

MICROWAVE

Electromagnetic waves with a frequency of 300 MHz – 300 GHz are classified as microwaves. More than just a means by which we cook popcorn, microwaves have long been used in telecommunications and broadcasting. Radar uses microwave radiation for applications such as air traffic control, weather prediction, and speed limit enforcement.

LIGHT

This is the portion of the electromagnetic spectrum that is visible to the human eye. However, other bands of the spectrum are often referred to as different forms of light. For example, infrared radiation is referred to as infrared light. Although it is not visible, it can be felt as heat. Stars and other hot objects in space emit ultraviolet radiation. UV waves are what cause our skin to burn. The frequency for infrared light is 10^{13} – 10^{14} Hz. The frequency for ultraviolet light is 10^{15} – 10^{16} Hz.

X-RAYS

While commonly associated with medical technology, hot gasses in our universe also emit X-rays with a frequency range between 30×10^{16} Hz – 3×10^{19} Hz.

GAMMA-RAYS

Radioactive materials emit gamma-rays. Some sources, like our universe, are natural while others, such as nuclear power plants, are manmade. The frequency range is 10^{20} Hz – 10^{24} Hz.

TECHNOLOGY

Technological devices appear at all levels of the EM spectrum. AM and FM radios, ultrasound, and TV broadcast all use the Radio Spectrum. Mobile phones, wireless data devices, and radar all use the Microwave Spectrum. Bio-imaging, security screening, remote control devices, lamps, and dental curing use the Light Spectrum, including infrared, visible, and ultraviolet. Medical x-rays and baggage screening use the X-ray spectrum. PET imaging uses the Gamma spectrum.

MANMADE VS. NATURE

As we can see from the previous examples, manmade devices and Mother Nature alike produce electromagnetic waves.

Even if we were to live in a remote part of the earth away from what are termed modern conveniences, we would still be impacted by electromagnetic frequencies.

◊ TWENTY THREE ◊

WHERE CAN I GO FOR HELP?

THE World Health Organization (WHO) recognizes this condition and terms it Electromagnetic Hypersensitivity (EHS). Officials in Sweden and the UK also recognize EMF Sensitivity. However, like many other complex conditions, professionals in the United States are slower than the rest of the world to recognize EMF Sensitivity as a real problem. As a result, it is difficult to find information and support, and much of what is out there is either incomplete, a scam, part of a conspiracy theory, or just plain inaccurate.

To make matters worse, many physicians advise their patients that the condition is purely psychological and recommend psychotherapy. To be fair, I imagine many physicians become frustrated when a number of therapies prove ineffective and they are left seeking non-physical causes. This is why keeping a journal can be helpful.

Because EMF Sensitivity is not widely accepted at this time, the burden of treatment falls to the patient. As an alternative practitioner suffering from EMF Sensitivity myself, I have experienced this first hand. Once I realized what was causing my symptoms, I sought non-invasive and non-pharmaceutical remedies that were low-cost and easily available.

All the therapies I have provided in this book are ones I discovered on my own and tried myself. They have been effective in reducing and/or eliminating the symptoms of EMF Sensitivity. I suggest that those who believe they are suffering from this condition try a variety of options and customize a program that helps them live more comfortably.

I think it is important to involve your family physician if you have been working with him or her to try and resolve your symptoms. If he or she is not supportive, I suggest seeking someone who is. This could be an open-minded family practitioner, an alternative medicine practitioner, or someone trained in environmental illness and/or multiple chemical sensitivities.

Under no circumstances should anyone quit taking medications without consulting a physician. Even if you are able to eliminate all your symptoms with a non-pharmaceutical remedy, your body needs to be weaned from medications under appropriate supervision in order to avoid serious health consequences.

I advise that people be wary of information available on the Internet. There are many individuals all too willing to take advantage of someone who may be suffering and feeling desperate enough to try anything and to pay anything to find relief. I implore people to be vigilant against scams and fraud.

Every treatment must be tailored to the individual and one may need to alternate a variety of treatments in order to find optimal relief. Also, not every treatment will necessarily work all the time. If there is a sudden increase in EMF emissions for some reason, the remedy may be rendered less effective.

Again, I point out that the only guaranteed treatment I am aware of is leaving the area of EMF exposure completely.

In closing this chapter I would like to pass along some wisdom. Some is ancient and some was given to me by my parents and grandparents.

Know thyself.

The Oracle at Delphi had it right. You really need to be aware of your body and to understand your health if you are to successfully maneuver your way through the muddied waters of EMF Sensitivity. Be aware of your natural rhythms; how your body and mood change with the seasons, under what circumstances you become more tired or achy, and what outside factors influence your well-being.

Finally, as my parents and grandparents repeatedly advised me throughout my growing years:

Never let anyone talk you into anything you aren't in agreement with; especially regarding your health. No one knows your body the way you do, not even a doctor. If you don't feel comfortable with something the doctor suggests, don't be afraid to get a second opinion. Pay attention and listen to your instincts.

Unfortunately, in our modern times people are too quick to believe that the specialist is the expert when it comes to their health. This simply isn't true. My parents had it right; no one knows our bodies the way we do. We need to look at our relationship with health care practitioners as a partnership. We need to take full responsibility for our health decisions including any tests, diagnosis, and treatments. This is particularly true when it comes to EMF Sensitivity.

Do yourself a favor; keep a journal.

◊ TWENTY FOUR ◊

How Do I Treat EMF Sensitivity?

THERE is no cure for EMF Sensitivity. However, there are steps one can take to mitigate and/or eliminate symptoms and significantly improve the quality of life. The following is a list from my own toolkit. I have personally tested every one and found most to be effective in lessening the severity of symptoms or eliminating them altogether. The ones that haven't worked as well for me are still included because they helped others who suffer symptoms as a result of EMF Sensitivity.

METALS

By far, the most effective remedy I have found has been direct exposure to copper, silver, and jeweler's brass. These metals insulate from the EMFs, resulting in a huge reduction of symptom severity, and in some cases, eliminating them altogether. The easiest way to accomplish this insulation is to wear jewelry made from these materials. The effect appears to be cumulative, so the more jewelry, the better.

The combination of copper, brass, and silver is individual. My husband wears a bracelet of silver and brass while mine are various combinations of the three metals. A friend gets tremendous relief from simply wearing two bracelets, one from copper and one from silver. Interestingly, he borrowed the copper one from his father who had been using it for its ability to eliminate arthritis pain.

I also have the silver necklace with its charms of copper, brass, and silver. I had hoped that by wearing the metals closer to my head I would alleviate the dizziness I was feeling. My theory was that by applying the metals closer to where the symptoms were manifesting I would be able to target them specifically. I successfully improved respiratory function and noticed a slight but still beneficial reduction in the vertigo symptoms.

I suggest that you experiment and tailor the solution to your own unique needs. The effect should be noticeable fairly quickly. While I got positive results the moment I put the bracelets on, others noticed improvement after an hour or two. The improvement in respiratory function from the necklace took a little longer to notice but the metallic content in the small charms is less than that of the bracelets.

The feedback regarding the benefits of the bracelets has been consistently positive. The most common improvement has been reduction and/or elimination of fatigue. In my own situation, in addition to a surge of energy, I no longer had burning, watery eyes, a runny nose, nausea, heartburn, or skin irritation. I also noticed an elimination of mood swings and an elimination of the depression and despair.

Don't be concerned if you notice green coloring on your skin or if your veins appear to be larger and closer to the surface. It does not necessarily mean you are wearing cheap jewelry. I believe it's a sign that the metals, particularly the copper, are doing their job.

I have observed that since wearing the bracelets my nails have become amazingly healthy, growing much faster than before and no longer breaking. I have not made any changes in my diet so I can only conclude that there is some correlation between the bracelets and the improved health of my nails.

You don't have to spend a lot of money on this remedy. A quick search on the Internet will show that copper, silver, and brass jewelry comes in all price ranges. The bracelets I found at the local New Age store are beautiful and very reasonably priced. I purchased the necklace charms from the Internet but I already knew that for me, a combination of all three metals was best. I recommend finding a local retailer, at least initially, so you can experience direct contact with the metals and find which ones work best for you.

MIRRORS

Heavy sliding mirrored doors have also made a difference. We kept our telecommunications and home office equipment behind them and when they were closed, any emissions from the equipment, particularly the laser printer, were effectively blocked.

The copper and silver in the reflective coating acts as an effective insulator. Closet doors made from wood cannot achieve the same relief. If you decide to install a mirrored closet door, I advise choosing a heavier one of good quality. I believe it will provide a higher level of shielding. Be sure that the source of problematic EMFs is located behind these doors and that they remain closed.

UNPLUG AND RELOCATE

The next most effective remedy I discovered took a little experimenting and research but was well worth it; it's one of the simplest.

Some of the smallest appliances require the most electricity. As you add devices, the power load increases and the likelihood of power leakage increases due to the electrical system approaching its maximum specification. In other words, too many electronic devices plugged into one room can be an incredible draw of current for your home or office.

Combine that with the numerous power strips needed for so many appliances and you have a recipe for an EMF nightmare. Fortunately, it's incredibly easy to fix.

First, evaluate what electronics really need to be located in the same place. If any of them can be moved to another location, do it. Spread them out. Additionally, try to reallocate the way the remaining ones are plugged in so that the power cords are not piled on top of each other. Do not fill up every single port on a power strip if you don't have to. Add an additional power strip across the room and move some of the appliances over to that one.

After moving a wireless printer to another part of our home and disconnecting the speakers that were hooked up to my computer, the symptoms I'd been suffering completely vanished. It took a little experimenting to figure out which devices were causing an issue but the research and relocation was incredibly effective. All it took was a little time and not-so-heavy lifting.

MINERAL SUPPLEMENTS

Research shows that copper is essential for energy and respiratory function. I have had consistent feedback that those who added a mineral supplement experienced an improvement in symptoms; particularly energy. Many multi-vitamin formulas already contain minerals, including copper, so check the labels to ensure you aren't taking too much. The RDA lists the daily value for Copper at 2mg.

SALT

It was my experience that immersion in bath water with a high saline content offered relief. Derek, who is also an experienced sailor, pointed out that salt water is one of the best blockers of EM waves; especially in the radio spectrum. It is also very conductive, unlike tap water.

I also felt noticeable relief when I held the salt stones that are used in salt lamps. I actually have a salt lamp in my office. It gives off an ambient light and I believe it helps absorb EM waves.

EXERCISE

I noticed that I felt much better after exercising. This was particularly true if I was having difficulty breathing due to EMF exposure. The moment I noticed that particular symptom increasing in severity, I would get moving. Pretty much any physical exercise did the trick, including brisk walking, running, lifting weights, yard work, even housework.

SAFE ROOM

I discovered that certain rooms in my home provided additional relief from symptoms. They are rooms that are free of any electronics other than reading lamps. Of course, some people could be sensitive to the EMFs emitted by lamps and would need to remove them from whatever space they choose to make into a safe room. A bedroom is well suited as a safe room although I am aware that many people keep televisions there. In order to make that space truly electronics-free, the TV would have to go. I would also suggest swapping out an alarm clock that plugs in with one that is operated on a battery or even an old-fashioned wind up alarm clock.

CHEWING GUM

Although it is one of the more temporary solutions since the positive effect is present only while actually chewing the gum, this remedy completely eliminated the health symptoms felt when exposed to the problematic EMFs. It also worked within the first minute of chewing; practically instantaneously.

FOOD

Good nutrition is always a sound idea but even more important when the body is under intense stress. EMF Sensitivity definitely taxes both the mind and body. The adrenal system is overburdened as the body tries to deal with the symptoms and the mind tries to reconcile fighting an invisible enemy.

In my own situation, the constant stress led to cravings for carbohydrates; the so-called comfort foods. Because my metabolism performs much better on a diet higher in protein, this led to weight gain. I stepped up my workout routine and cut calories to no avail.

Interestingly, I observed that when I left the area for extended periods of time, even on vacations when most of us pay little attention to what we eat, I lost a great deal of weight. When I returned, the cravings, and the weight, came back. Once I discovered the bracelets, I was able to regain balance, eliminate carbohydrate cravings, and lose the unwanted pounds.

My belief is that overstressed adrenals put the body into physiological survival mode. Not only are people likely to crave comfort foods notoriously high in sugar and fat, but also the body's own metabolism may work against us by keeping weight on as part of that survival effort.

Keep a journal and tweak your diet until you find an eating pattern that is in harmony with your body. Eliminate any foods that make you feel worse.

ALCOHOL

Alcohol is a depressant that affects brain waves and motor function. People who drink can experience vision disturbances, dizziness, memory impairment, and changes in mood, including depression. These are all symptoms associated with EMF Sensitivity. Because of this, drinking alcohol while impacted by EMFs can result in a significant increase in symptom intensity. Quite frankly, any positive effects associated with social drinking might be outweighed by how sick you feel.

Beginning in April 2008, after my symptoms intensified in number and severity, I began to crave certain alcoholic beverages; specifically, red wine and margaritas. I believe this sudden craving was similar to craving carbohydrates. My adrenals were overstressed and the relaxing effect that alcohol offered was a way to counter the effect; at least in theory. Unfortunately, after even one or two of these beverages, the symptoms intensified, including dizziness, depression and hopelessness. In fact, I felt so sick that I quit drinking entirely whenever in an area of EMF exposure.

However, in my situation, the effects were geographic and by simply leaving the area of exposure, were eliminated.

On days when the symptoms of EMF Sensitivity are particularly bad I feel as if I'm hung over even if I haven't had any alcohol. I have heard similar feedback from others who have sensitivity to electromagnetic frequencies.

CAFFEINE

Just as alcohol acts as a depressant, caffeine acts as a stimulant. During times of severe fatigue, caffeine has been a true lifesaver for me. However, there is a drawback. Caffeine puts stress on the adrenal glands, which are already overburdened due to EMF Sensitivity.

I have also observed a relationship between dizziness and increased caffeine intake. However, since the severe fatigue was outright debilitating at times, I felt the temporary increase in dizziness was more than worth it. My suggestion is to carefully manage caffeine intake and be sure to drink plenty of water.

TEA

The brainwave changes brought about by exposure to problematic EMFs meant that medications and vibrational therapies were no longer effective for me. Herbal teas, however, continued to have therapeutic value. The key to remember is that herbal teas are taken for specific uses. In other words, they won't bring immunity from EMF triggers but they will help support overall health.

For example, pau d'arco and red clover tea are excellent blood purifiers, whereas dandelion root and nettles teas are great tonics for the kidneys. I used various teas to help strengthen my immune system, which was taking a constant beating, and got good results.

DETOX

There is information that suggests detoxifying the body brings symptomatic relief. This could be due to strengthening the body and the immune system or it could be that what was thought of as EMF Sensitivity is really multiple chemical sensitivities. While detoxification has merit and can benefit overall health, I can't stress enough that it should be done under the supervision of someone familiar with various methods. I also advise against detoxification if someone is very ill or weak. The process of removing toxins from the body is energy intensive and can often leave someone feeling worse before they are able to feel the benefits. However, it makes sense to see where in your diet and lifestyle you can make various improvements, such as quitting smoking, cutting back on drinking alcohol or caffeine, and adding an exercise routine.

MEDICATIONS

In attempting to address the myriad of symptoms I'd had while living in the San Francisco Bay Area, I tried a number of therapies, both traditional and alternative. None of the medications associated with these therapies worked. In fact, it got to a point where even simple over-the-counter medicines such as aspirin were no longer effective. I believe this is because of the way my brainwaves were being affected.

In the summer of 2008, I became aware that vibrational therapies had ceased to be effective. Since I am an alternative practitioner, I found this both alarming and disappointing. After decades of successfully using homeopathy, flower remedies, and acupuncture, I no longer found any relief. Apparently, the EMF-induced changes in my cells were overriding the therapeutic effects of these therapies.

In my personal experience, as long as the body is exposed to the problematic EMFs, medications, both natural and pharmaceutical, are rendered ineffective. However, once away from the source of problematic EMFs, the therapies seemed to work just fine.

BENADRYL©

While living in the Bay Area I tried various allergy medications to relieve symptoms but experienced a minimum of relief. The exception was when I applied topical Benadryl to my skin for the relief of the mysterious itching. After relocating I tested oral Benadryl and found it quite effective at relieving symptoms associated with EMF Sensitivity. I believe the body, in its attempt to cope with the onslaught caused by EMF exposure, releases histamines as part of the immune response. The antihistamines in Benadryl effectively calm this immune response, regardless of the cause.

However, I want to reiterate that EMF Sensitivity is not an allergy. Repeated and extended exposure actually makes it worse. There are no shots to increase tolerance. To write it off as a simple allergy , in my opinion, is a mistake.

And while it's great to have another therapy, I want to advise caution. A side effect of Benadryl is drowsiness. I suggest careful implementation of this therapy and using it in conjunction with other treatments, not as the primary one.

SUPPLEMENTS

Shortly after we moved to our East Bay home, I began to take vitamin C and magnesium on a daily basis. This decision was unconscious and was not, to my knowledge, related to any specific condition. Interestingly, I came across a reference to these two nutrients in a study of EMF Sensitivity done at the Environmental Health Center in Dallas, Texas[29]. Patients who had had a severe response to EMF exposure were treated with an IV containing vitamin C and magnesium. I can only surmise that on an unconscious level I understood that these two supplements would provide some sort of nutritional support even though at the time I was unaware of what was causing the symptoms.

I happen to believe in cellular intelligence and have seen plenty of examples of the body instinctively knowing what it needed nutritionally by craving certain foods and beverages.[30]

As a general rule I think taking a multi-vitamin and mineral supplement is a good idea; especially when the body is under stress and one's diet is out of balance. When it comes to nutritional supplements, one can choose from food-based, natural, or synthetic. In my experience, no one is necessarily better than another.

Everyone's metabolism is unique and what works for one person may not for another. I don't believe that higher priced vitamins are necessarily better than less expensive and, in my experience, prescription-based are not any better than over-the-counter. My suggestion is to try a variety of brands and see if you notice any difference.

It's also not a bad idea to periodically give your body a rest from nutritional supplements and even to rotate brands and the supplements themselves. If you're worried about the loss of nutrition, try juicing. It's a wonderful way to get vitamins and minerals.

MUSIC

It has been my experience that the sound waves associated with certain types of music provide interference to the problematic frequencies, alleviating some of the symptoms. In my own case, music was most effective in combating the feelings of depression and hopelessness that occurred during times of high EMF emissions. I also experienced a surge in energy that would last between thirty minutes and three hours after listening to the helpful tunes.

I did notice that it was a very specific beat associated with certain heavy metal songs that made a difference for me. Interestingly, I didn't need to like the song for it to be effective. As long as it had that specific beat I obtained significant improvement.

I tested classic rock, hip-hop, and a variety of other types of music and none of them accomplished the same relief as heavy metal and hard rock. I suggest spending time testing several songs by various artists.

Feedback from others has been consistent with my own experience in that music with a strong beat, such as dance music or rock, has the best effect.

If possible, organize these songs and have them available for mobility. A portable music player, such as an iPod, is ideally suited for this.

I have over a dozen songs to choose from and have found that after approximately four, my symptoms have lessened significantly or disappeared entirely. While I don't condone excessive volume, during times of intense symptom severity, I personally find relief comes more quickly when the music is loud. However, as soon as I feel better, I reduce the volume.

NOISE CANCELING HEADPHONES

I have found that within minutes of activating noise canceling headphones, feelings of despair associated with certain EMFs disappear. The longer the noise canceling headphones are activated the longer the effect will last after turning them off.

I also noticed that they eliminate the symptoms associated with exposure to fluorescent lighting. When I wear them in a grocery store, for instance, I do not experience the difficulty concentrating and fatigue I would if I were not wearing them.

Although I personally use the Bose noise canceling headphones, there are other brands. I suggest you experiment in order to find which works best for you.

MEDITATION

Meditation can bring peace of mind and stress relief, both invaluable when suffering from health issues.

For years I had been using a form of meditation, known as the Silva method, that teaches relaxation and problem solving, primarily utilizing the alpha state[31]. I noticed that beginning in April 2008, when the network infrastructure in our neighborhood had been upgraded, it was almost impossible for me to achieve and maintain a meditative state.

This was a sudden change, and I believe related to the EMF emissions that I am sensitive to and how they affect my brain waves. I tried countering this difficulty by listening to recorded tones associated with the Silva program that are meant to help achieve the alpha state and deepen relaxation while meditating. I got mixed results.

I also noticed to my dismay that any visualization I attempted as part of the Silva Method's mental programming went completely haywire. I had been successfully using this method since 2000 so I have to conclude that the sudden inability to successfully visualize and program for problem solving was directly related to the negative effect of the EMFs.

I have gotten similar feedback from others who suffer from EMF Sensitivity.

LOCATION

Well, this one may seem a little obvious but I won't take anything for granted. The single most effective remedy that works every time, without fail, is to get away from the source of the trouble; whatever is emitting the problematic frequency.

If someone is fortunate, that may simply mean moving the printer out of their office. Some people have gone so far as to give up their cell phones or other personal devices.

My experience has been that those who wear the jewelry are able to continue interacting with technology without difficulty, even when that is the source of the problematic frequency.

But what if the problematic EMFs are not technological in origin? For those of us sensitive to EMFs from Mother Nature, only relocating to a more hospitable environment will bring complete relief. If relocating is not an option there are still things you can do to relieve symptoms.

Before we relocated to an area away from fault lines, my family took frequent day trips to areas away from our home so I could experience relief. San Francisco, where there are no fault lines, and short vacations to old silver and copper mining towns, were the most common. I observed that for every eight hours I was completely away from the sources of the problematic EMFs, I could spend approximately eighteen hours back in their proximity before I was severely affected.

You need to consider your quality of life. How bad are the symptoms? How disruptive are they for you and your family? Only you can decide.

There is no one right answer.

PART III

CASE STUDIES

◊ TWENTY FIVE ◊

WILL THESE THERAPIES HELP ME?

GAIL was tired of being tired. After a thorough physical including relevant blood tests ruled out any health issues, she consulted me. She complained of nausea, dizziness, dragging, difficulty concentrating and exhaustion. She also mentioned having gained weight even though she exercised and watched her caloric intake.

A history revealed that she had been tired all of her life but had attributed the cause to allergies. Additionally, for years she believed she suffered from Fibromyalgia or Chronic Fatigue Syndrome.

After careful questioning I began to suspect she had electromagnetic sensitivity to the EMFs from fault lines. I must admit I was a bit surprised. I would have thought that, as a west coast native, she would be immune to any sensitivity related directly to the geologic uniqueness of her surroundings. However, I couldn't ignore the fact that her symptoms were incredibly close to what I had experienced, including a random pattern with no easily discernable cause.

I asked her to keep a journal so I could compare the data against earthquake information on the USGS website. Sure enough, I observed a relationship between her symptoms and the dates and times of earthquakes, including a reduction in severity or total elimination of some of them after a quake occurred.

At this point I shared my suspicions with Gail. Needless to say, she was surprised by the idea that EMFs from fault lines could be responsible for her complaints.

"This is the last place I would have looked."

By and large her biggest complaint was chronic fatigue.

I suggested that she try the bracelets and see if they made a difference. I told her where she could purchase them and suggested she spend time trying different ones to determine which, if any, had the most positive impact.

Her response came quickly. She excitedly told me that she had purchased two bracelets and almost immediately noticed an increase in energy. She felt great. Her mental clarity had returned, she was energetic and she woke up feeling normal with energy.

"It has been wonderful."

At this point I suggested that she take a daily mineral supplement. I explained that since studies showed that copper is responsible for energy as well as healthy respiratory function, she might experience additional benefits from taking it internally. Her feedback was quick and positive. She felt much better and more energetic after taking a mineral supplement that included copper.

At one point Gail contacted me to inquire about new symptoms. She had been feeling irritable, grouchy, and stressed in the hours and days prior to an earthquake on nearby faults. I confirmed that yes, mood changes such as these were symptoms associated with electromagnetic sensitivity, and that since she experienced them when the EMF emissions from the fault lines were higher, it made perfect sense that she felt them when she did. I suggested she try purchasing another bracelet to see if it helped reduce or eliminate these symptoms.

Over time, I continued to hear positive feedback from Gail. She had purchased a new watch with a stainless steel band and continued to wear the bracelets. She continued to experience higher levels of energy, and pointed out that she was *groovin' around really fast*.

◊ ◊ ◊ ◊ ◊

CAROLYN, a CEO in the Midwest, strongly suspected something about her home was making her sick.

155

Shortly after moving in she began to experience headaches, allergy symptoms, and a constant fatigue. She also suffered difficulty concentrating.

After a thorough medical exam including blood tests and an MRI ruled out any health issues she asked me if I had any ideas.

During our interview I learned that a geologic fault line ran very close to her home. I explained about the relationship between EMFs and fault lines and told her about the bracelets. I further explained about the relationship between supplemental copper and respiratory function and energy levels. I suggested she try purchasing a bracelet or two, being sure to spend time trying a variety on and seeing how she felt. I also suggested she add a mineral supplement to her diet.

After several weeks I got a note from Carolyn. She had located a shop that sold the bracelets and purchased two. Almost immediately she felt a surge in energy and her mental clarity improved significantly.

Another month went by and I got another note. Carolyn said that she felt really good. In fact she wondered where she was getting all the energy she had. She told me that she still wore bracelets fashioned from all three metals as they seemed to feel the best.

◊ ◊ ◊ ◊ ◊

BRIAN, a school teacher living in the south, was scheduled for an MRI. He had been suffering vertigo on and off for years and in the previous months it had become so severe it had turned his life inside out.

"It has been a nightmare."

He went on to describe that he had always been healthy so this had been a complete shock to get used to. He had undergone extensive and invasive testing and although his doctor had ruled out obvious causes such as an inner ear infection, he had not found any explanation. He scheduled Brian for an MRI scan to learn more.

Brian also complained of nausea and exhaustion. He said the loss of concentration he experienced was incredible.

"I am there but out in space. Like being on some drug that slows the brain down...rather an odd experience. I am to the point where it is happening seriously every three weeks. That time frame is getting shorter."

When I heard those words I immediately suspected electromagnetic sensitivity. I remembered that in my own case I felt as if someone had poured molasses on my brain and as if I'd been given drugs that slowed my brain down. It was a horrible feeling.

Because of my previous research regarding fault zone locations across the country I was pretty confident this wasn't what was affecting Brian; there were none anywhere close to his home. As a result, I focused on the more traditionally accepted cause of electromagnetic sensitivity; technology.

Careful questioning revealed that the onset of the vertigo coincided with the installation of wireless technology in his home. In the beginning the incidents were few and far between.

"Nothing major."

Then at the start of the year he noticed an increase in symptoms. Further questioning revealed that this is when he had acquired a new mobile personal technology device. As time went on and he continued to use the new technology more often, his symptoms increased in intensity and frequency to the point where they were debilitating.

My heart went out to Brian. I completely understood what he was going through. I felt badly about the invasive tests he had been subjected to as they had more than taken a toll on his well-being.

I told him what I thought was happening and why. I gave him as thorough an explanation as possible, and related the success I'd had with bracelets made from copper, silver, and brass.

"Well I put a silver band on and a thick copper bracelet on the other arm…laid down for 2 hrs and it's weird no spins…"

Twelve hours later I heard from him again.

"So far still ok…rather unreal…bands are copper and silver seems to be doing the trick…"

He went on to add *"I of course am skeptical because of everything I have been through to date…but can't dispute the no spins…Really hope the relief continues…it has brought me to my knees as far as accomplishing simple daily functions…"*

I continued to get positive feedback.

"Still feel no spins to this hour…I am going to be out and about trying a few things I have had to cut out for the past few months and see if my spins will crank up…I hate to push a good thing but might as well find out…Still rather shocked but with a happy smile on my face…I'll keep you updated today."

A few days later I heard more good news.

"Still no problems little woozy but no spins…Can't Thank you enough."

Brian was scheduled for an MRI, a relatively new diagnostic test that uses a powerful magnetic field to align the nuclear magnetization of hydrogen atoms in water in the body. Radio Frequency fields are used to alter the alignment of this magnetization, causing the hydrogen nuclei to produce a rotating magnetic field detectable by the scanner. The signal can be manipulated by additional magnetic fields to build up enough information to construct an image of the body.

I was concerned that due to the magnetic field involved in the test Brian would experience a temporary relapse in symptoms. At the same time I felt confident that once he put the bracelets back on any symptoms would reduce and eventually disappear. As it turned out the test went well and he didn't experience any discomfort.

"Doing fine…Hope it is because of the metal…Actually got out of the house again today…this is the first time within a couple of weeks I have felt normal…trying to build back up to a routine…"

Recent communication with Brian confirmed he is still wearing the bracelets and he is still free from symptoms. However, he did relate that he had experienced a short return of the vertigo but his doctor, suspecting it was from an inner ear infection, prescribed a course of antibiotics. This resolved the vertigo and he is again free of symptoms. He told me that he wears four bracelets; two are solid silver, one is brass and copper, and one is solely copper. He also has a thin gold chain around his neck.

The above examples illustrate that the treatments for EMF Sensitivity consistently provide relief to a variety of symptoms, regardless of the source of the problematic EMFs. The treatments work for men and women alike, regardless of age or location. All three individuals continue to utilize technology in their daily lives without any difficulty.

It is my hope that people who suffer from EMF Sensitivity will take heart from these examples and will be inspired to experiment with the therapies I've provided.

PART IV

POINTS TO PONDER

◊ TWENTY SIX ◊

EMF SENSITIVITY, CFS AND FIBROMYALGIA

WHILE researching symptoms of EMF Sensitivity, I made a startling observation. The symptoms for EMF Sensitivity, Chronic Fatigue Syndrome, and Fibromyalgia were identical. Even before drawing a side-by-side comparison of symptoms, however, I had begun to suspect that Chronic Fatigue Syndrome was, in reality, EMF Sensitivity. I was able to strengthen my hypothesis following feedback from a friend.

After ruling out medical problems and eliminating nutritional deficiencies, I had suggested she try the bracelets to see if she could find any relief from her symptoms. I was pleased to learn she felt much better after wearing them and that she had found a great deal more energy. One of her comments in particular got my attention:

"...all those years I thought that I might have had Fibromyalgia or Chronic Fatigue Syndrome..."

In light of the information illustrated in *Table 2*, I would love to see people who believe they suffer from Chronic Fatigue Syndrome and Fibromyalgia take a closer look and see if perhaps what they are really suffering from is EMF Sensitivity. I think it would be wonderful to be free of medications and to find relief from simpler, less invasive solutions.

I would like to stress that such an investigation should be taken with the guidance of a health professional.

Table 2: EMF Sensitity v. CFS v. Fibromyalgia

EMF Sensitivity	Chronic Fatigue Syndrome	Fibromyalgia
Fatigue	Fatigue	Fatigue
Exhaustion	Exhaustion that lasts more than 24 hours after physical exercise	Extreme fatigue
Problems with memory	Loss of memory	Memory impairment
Concentration issues	Loss of concentration	Cognitive impairment
Pain that is typically in the muscles or even the joints	Unexplained muscle pain and pain that moves from one joint to another	Muscle twitches and weakness
Mild to severe headaches	New type of headache, pattern or severity	Headaches
Toothaches	Jaw pain	TMJ, jaw pain
Problems in sleep	Unrefreshing sleep	Sleep disorders
Swelling and itching in facial area	Bloating	Myofascial pain
Allergies	Allergies & sensitivities	Cold symptoms
Gastric problems	Abdominal pain	Abdominal pain
Extreme dizziness, balance problems, and in severe cases, loss of consciousness	Dizziness, balance problems, or fainting	Dizziness
Irregular heartbeat	Irregular heartbeat	Stabbing pain in chest and rib cage
Ringing and clicking in ears	Earache	Ringing in ears and ear pain
Nausea with or w/o vomiting	Nausea	Nausea
Depression, irritability, mood swings	Depression, irritability, anxiety and panic attacks	Depression, anxiety
Difficulty breathing	Shortness of breath	Trouble breathing
Tingling, burning, pins and needles sensations	Tingling sensations	

◊ TWENTY SEVEN ◊

EMF Sensitivity and Multiple Chemical Sensitivity

EARLY in my research I came across an article that proclaimed there is no such thing as EMF Sensitivity; that the symptoms were actually a result of Multiple Chemical Sensitivity (MCS). I don't agree with this. I have never been sensitive to perfumes or detergents or any of the chemical triggers suspected of wreaking havoc in someone with this condition. What I found interesting was the similarity the symptoms of MSC and EMF sensitivity. Refer to *Table 3*.

Table 3: EMF Sensitity v. MCS

EMF Sensitivity	Multiple Chemical Sensitivity
Fatigue	Extreme Fatigue
Exhaustion	Lethargy
Problems with memory	Poor memory
Concentration issues	Poor concentration
Pain that is typically in the muscles or even the joints	Muscle and joint pain
Mild to severe headaches	Headaches, migraines
Toothaches	Sinus problems
Problems in sleep	Sleeping problems
Skin rashes, itching	Skin rashes, itching
Runny nose	Runny nose
Gastric problems	Digestive upset
Extreme dizziness, balance problems, and in severe cases, loss of consciousness	Vertigo, dizziness
Ringing and clicking in ears	Earache
Nausea with or without vomiting	Nausea
Difficulty breathing	Wheezing, breathlessness
Watery, burning eyes	Burning, stinging eyes

Even more startling was the same lack of understanding by the medical community. Like EMF Sensitivity, MCS was considered an unexplainable phenomenon and was met with great skepticism.

It did not fit the profile of true allergies so there was no known understanding of causes or the process by which it acted on the body.

Because only a small percentage of individuals suffered symptoms and it differed from one patient to the next, treatments offered by the medical community were often ineffective or inappropriate.

The similarities between the two conditions are startling, and, I believe, worthy of a second look.

◇ TWENTY EIGHT ◇

EMF SENSITIVITY, ADD, AND ADHD

ALTHOUGH the symptomology between EMF Sensitivity and ADD or ADHD is not completely identical like with CFS, Fibromyalgia, and MCS, I still think that many cases of Attention Deficit Disorder (ADD) and Attention Deficit Hypersensitivity Disorder (ADHD) are really EMF Sensitivity.

Two of the major symptoms of ADD and ADHD are inattention and inability to concentrate. I can attest from personal experience that when the symptoms from my EMF Sensitivity are severe, I feel as if I've been given a tranquilizer. Not only do I have difficulty concentrating, I am in a daze. People have to repeatedly ask even the simplest questions before I am able to answer. I have difficulty completing the most mundane tasks, such as deciding what to eat.

After discovering the bracelets, these symptoms were significantly reduced. However, within minutes of entering a grocery store with fluorescent lighting or when I am in an area where there is a fault line, the symptoms return, and the longer the exposure, the worse they become.

In September 2009, we attended a Renaissance Festival. To my dismay, I found that I was barely able to function. The simple act of getting popcorn at a booth turned into a monumental effort because of an intense difficulty concentrating. It turns out the park where the festival was being held sits on a Bay Area fault line.

One CEO related that while in the presence of problematic EMFs, his concentration was so affected he had difficulty signing his name on some business contracts. Additionally, when he did sign, he mistakenly used an older signature that he had not utilized in years.

According to the Centers for Disease Control and Prevention, the number of people diagnosed with ADHD has increased by an average of 3% a year between 1997 and 2005.[32] During that same time period, thanks to advances in technology and a reduction in manufacturing costs, almost every school in the country put computers in the classrooms, libraries, and other areas. Although there is no doubt that they are invaluable for enhancing the educational experience, I fear that the frequencies they give off are harming a percentage of the students exposed to them. Because the symptoms of EMF Sensitivity are similar to those of ADD and ADHD, I believe that the children affected by the problematic frequencies are misdiagnosed and worse, put on medication needlessly.

I am aware that most children undergo intensive testing and psychiatric evaluations as part of the process of accurately diagnosing ADD and ADHD. Indeed, while earning my bachelor's in holistic childcare I had a course, focused solely on ADD, in which the author of the textbook stressed the importance of accurate diagnostic procedures by an appropriately trained ADD specialist. However, given that the equipment used in testing gives off EMFs, not to mention the fact that just about every doctor's office contains computers, printers, fluorescent lighting and networking equipment, how can we be sure that the results are being interpreted correctly?

It is estimated that between 3 and 5 percent of American children are affected by ADHD. Worldwide polls have revealed that between 1.5 and 3 percent of the population is EMF sensitive. The comparison is compelling, and, I believe, warrants further study. It would be a tragedy to unnecessarily medicate a healthy child.

◊ TWENTY NINE ◊

EMF Sensitivity and SAD

AS I was preparing to go to press, I discovered a possible link between EMF Sensitivity and Seasonal Affective Disorder (SAD). This link, an over-production of histamine, may turn out to be the key to understanding EMF Sensitivity.

From the time I was a teen, I suffered terrible migraines during thunderstorm season. California weather patterns are significantly different than those in the Midwest, so this wasn't a problem I faced while living there. However, after moving to Colorado, I found myself again facing health issues from storm systems. In particular, I noticed that in addition to a headache, in the hours before a storm system moved through our area, I suffered a mild to moderate depression, and a sense of hopelessness.

I knew that, like the fault lines, these storm systems put out ultra-low EMFs. I also knew that I was sensitive to these ultra-low frequencies, and suffered a variety of negative health symptoms because of them. Unfortunately, understanding wasn't enough, since I was unable to completely eliminate this disturbing symptom.

What was particularly puzzling was that the metal jewelry eliminated headaches associated with storm system EMFs, and depression associated with fault line EMFs, but was ineffective in resolving the depression caused by storm system EMFs. Because I lived in a part of the country where these storm systems were a frequent occurrence, I began to feel an urgent need to find a remedy that would eliminate this symptom. The alternative, spending half my time feeling depressed, wasn't an option.

I had tried all but one of the remedies in an attempt to eliminate the negative mood changes associated with storm systems. I did not try Benadryl. Even if it did provide relief, it caused drowsiness, so it was not a remedy I could take on a regular basis. I reviewed the various therapies and the principles upon which they worked, and found myself coming back to the Benadryl. I had long suspected that the symptoms of EMF Sensitivity resulted from an immune system response; the release of histamine. This would explain why EMF Sensitivity had so many commonalities with allergies. Benadryl is an antihistamine and it did resolve symptoms associated with EMF Sensitivity; backing up this theory.

While researching this angle, I stumbled upon some interesting observations. The symptoms of seasonal affective disorder are similar to those of EMF Sensitivity. There is also an overlap of symptoms between EMF Sensitivity and histadelia, a condition wherein there is an overproduction of histamine (See *Table 4*).

What was even more interesting was that histadelia was sometimes misdiagnosed as SAD. People who suffer from SAD tend to manifest symptoms during the fall and winter, when there is less sunshine and more cloud cover. I felt symptoms whenever there was intense cloud cover, such as when thunderstorms were moving through.

It didn't have to be raining for me to develop symptoms. It was the presence of numerous low-hanging clouds, as opposed to the higher fluffy ones that dot an otherwise clear sky that brought on the depression and sense of hopelessness. This cloud cover is similar to the weather patterns associated with seasonal affective disorder.

Table 4: EMF Sensitivity v. SAD v. Histadelia

EMF Sensitivity	Seasonal Affective Disorder	Histadelia
Fatigue	Loss of Energy	Fatigue
Depression	Depression	Depression
Headaches	Headaches	Headaches
Problems sleeping	Difficulty sleeping	Insomnia, problems sleeping
Weight gain	Weight gain	
Difficulty concentrating	Difficulty concentrating	
Craving carbohydrates	Craving carbohydrates	
Nausea		Unexplained nausea
Joint pain, swelling, stiffness		Joint pain, swelling, stiffness
Warm skin/fever		Warm skin
Runny nose		Allergic rhinitis
Watery eyes		Excessive tears
Excessive mucous		Excessive mucous
Muscle pain		Muscle pain

There is a high incidence of alcoholism among histadeliacs. Studies have shown that alcohol, and, red wine in particular, is anti-inflammatory. This is one of the properties of antihistamines, something that would be helpful in treating the overproduction of histamine.

Vitamin C and magnesium are among the supplements suggested for treating histadelia. Some doctors use this combination to treat symptoms of EMF Sensitivity.

L-Methionine is another supplement used in the treatment of histadelia. I have had positive results when using it to treat symptoms of EMF Sensitivity related to excessive cloud cover.

Studies have established relationships between nutritional levels of copper and zinc, and histadelia. Copper and zinc, albeit in a different form, are two of the most effective remedies I have found for treating EMF Sensitivity; probably not a coincidence.

◊ THIRTY ◊

WHAT DOES NATURE HAVE TO SAY?

WHILE researching the fact that electromagnetic energy affects the organisms living on this planet, I was astounded by the number of times US officials dismissed evidence accepted by scientists and professionals from all over the world, and documented as far back as 300 BC. I repeatedly saw the word *inconclusive* used by one *expert* or another.

In trying to understand why educated individuals would refute numerous studies done by scientists, physicists, and professionals from accredited universities, I considered everything from superstition, to lack of imagination, to outright stubbornness.

Dismissing all of the above, I focused instead on who *was* supporting these ideas, and where they were located. By far, the preponderance of them seemed to be in Asia; in particular, China. When I thought about why this was, I theorized that many of the citizens living in China continue to live an agricultural way of life and, as a result, are much more in tune with the environment than their counterparts from industrialized areas.

Because their livelihood may depend on the animals in their care, they had better know them to the extent that they can practically read their minds. If the failure or success of their crops depends on the weather, they'd better know how to read the skies as well as, if not better than a trained meteorologist. With so much at stake, in order to live in harmony with the world around them, they had certainly better have an intimate understanding of it.

As my father likes to say, *"You can't beat Mother Nature so you had better learn to respect her."*

While we're on the subject, why don't we see just what Mother Nature has to say about EMFs affecting her environment?

LARGE MAMMALS ARE SENSITIVE TO LOW FREQUENCY ELECTROMAGNETIC FIELDS.

In the March 16, 2009 issue of *Proceedings of the National Academy of Sciences*, researchers revealed that when away from the mild electromagnetic fields omitted by power lines, cows and deer herds aligned themselves along a north-south axis. However, when exposed to the EMFs, they pointed in different directions.

These findings constitute evidence for magnetic sensation in large mammals as well as evidence of an overt behavioral reaction to weak [extreme low-frequency magnetic fields] in vertebrates.[33]

BATS ARE SENSITIVE TO EMFS.

Although the reasons are not understood, bats are more vulnerable to collisions with wind turbines than birds. Researchers at the University of Aberdeen had long observed that bat activity in the vicinity of the Aberdeen Civil Air Traffic Control (ATC) radar station was reduced, in spite of the number of bat habitats close by. This led them to question whether the radio frequency (RF) radiation associated with the radar installation may elicit an aversive behavioral response in foraging bats.

Between June and September 2006, researchers obtained samplings at ten radar stations as part of a study to prove whether or not this was a valid hypothesis. Results revealed that bat activity was significantly reduced in areas where the habitats were exposed to EMF strength greater than 2 v/m when compared to sites registering EMF levels of zero.[34]

ANIMALS DETECT EMFs FROM FAULT LINES.

For centuries, significant changes in animal behavior prior to earthquakes have been observed. In 373 BC it was recorded that animals, including rats, snakes and weasels, deserted Helice in droves days before a quake devastated the Greek City. In 2003, a Japanese doctor released details of a study that indicated erratic behavior in dogs prior to earthquakes.

Prior to the 1994 Northridge, California earthquake, there were reports of dogs howling mysteriously, caged birds becoming restless, and nervous cats hiding. The same was true prior to the 1999 Greek and Turkish earthquakes.

In various countries around the globe there have been reports of animals behaving strangely prior to an earthquake. In May 2008, the AP reported that in the hours and days prior to a deadly earthquake, news of animals behaving oddly emerged throughout China. One province was overrun with toads days before it struck. At a zoo 600 miles from the epicenter, the animals began acting strangely in the hours before it hit. The zebras began banging their heads against the doors of their enclosures; the elephants swung their trunks wildly; lions were awake at times when they would normally be napping; and the peacocks screeched in unison as if in warning.

Although US officials tend to dismiss this phenomenon in spite of similar stories here, researchers in other countries, particularly those in China and Japan, continue to study and report on such findings. They hope to learn enough that they can utilize the changes in the animals' behavior as part of an early quake detection system.

WHAT'S GOING ON?

One theory reported by the National Geographic News was that the animals are able to detect electrical changes in the air or gas released from the Earth.[35] Since scientists around the globe have documented increased EMF output from fault lines in the hours and days prior to the earthquake, the exact times the animals' behavior becomes erratic, it is logical to conclude that the animals are being affected by the increased EMF output.

EARTHQUAKE WEATHER

The idea that a certain type of weather precedes earthquakes dates back to ancient Greece when Aristotle proposed that they were caused by winds trapped in subterranean caves. However, speak with Bay Area residents who clearly recall the 1989 Loma Prieta quake and you are very likely to hear a similar theory.

Interestingly, what they describe as earthquake weather sounds a lot like what Midwesterners call tornado weather, suggesting that something observable, if not unusual is going on.

One of the keys to validating this weather phenomenon may be in our skies.

Historical records from the ancient civilizations of China, India, and Rome suggest a correlation between certain cloud formations and earthquakes. The ancient Indian scholar, Brihat Samhita, noted extraordinary cloud formations that appeared prior to earthquakes. In December 2004, geophysicists in Henan, China noted that there was a gap in the clouds that precisely matched the location of the main fault in Southern Iran.[36] This gap stretched for hundreds of miles and was visible for hours, in the same place, even as the clouds around it continued to move. Sixty-nine days later, a deadly earthquake occurred. In 2005, a similar formation appeared sixty-four days prior to a magnitude 6 quake that shook the region.

NASA researcher Friedemann Freund demonstrated that when rocks are squeezed, positively charged ions form in the air above, suggesting an electromagnetic relationship of some sort exists and warrants further investigation. Thanks to satellite technology, researchers are able to continue studies of odd cloud formations in the vicinity of active fault zones in the days and weeks prior to earthquakes.

It would certainly appear that Mother Nature is coming out in support of EMF Sensitivity.

◊ THIRTY ONE ◊

EMFS AND PSI

WHILE researching and documenting various EMF cause and effect relationships I made some rather intriguing observations regarding electromagnetic energy and psychic abilities.

All my life I have had a highly developed sixth sense. In fact, shortly after moving to our East Bay home in 2005, I *received* an incredibly strong intuitive message that we needed to move away from the Bay Area. As we had just closed on our house less than a month before, I was far from eager to share this with Aaron. However, as I had coached him on not shooting the messenger when it came to such revelations long before we were married, I went ahead and relayed the information. Needless to say, he wasn't all too pleased. Especially when the only reason I could provide for why we needed to move was that some psychic feeling told me so.

However, not long after that day I began to feel ill. Fatigue was the first symptom, followed by a sense of hopelessness. I began to have difficulty concentrating and it wasn't long before I was facing an overwhelming progression of mysterious and seemingly unrelated symptoms.

At this same time, I noticed that my extra-sensory abilities had begun to disappear. Since they had been a part of my life since early childhood, I became quite alarmed and not a little unnerved by this development. In fact, there was one particularly eerie aspect that began to wreak havoc with my emotions.

Throughout my life, from the time I was five years old, I had been able to predict future events with startling accuracy. My premonitions often came through dreams, although it was not unusual for me to spontaneously become conscious of some event yet to happen. As a result, I had a heightened awareness of the world around me. Not long after moving into our East Bay home I realized that not only did I no longer have this ability, I could no longer sense any future at all.

I was pregnant at this point, and since I accessed my extra-sensory abilities primarily through my solar plexus, I theorized that in an effort to protect the growing baby from harmful outside energies, my body had shut and locked the door so to speak. However, when my abilities failed to return after my child was born I became concerned.

As time went on and I was still unable to see or feel any future for myself I began to wonder if that meant I was going to die soon; that on some unconscious level I knew something my conscious mind wasn't ready to acknowledge. This added a whole new dimension to the depression I was fighting. Knowing I was too young to feel so old and too healthy to feel so sick, I began to search for an explanation.

It soon became apparent that my clairvoyance wasn't the only ability I no longer had access to. It would seem that all of my psi abilities, including my strong sense of intuition, were, at the least significantly reduced, and at the worst, completely gone; an apparent casualty of the EMF Sensitivity.

Since I hadn't yet discovered that I was sensitive to electromagnetic frequencies at that point in time, I simply had no idea what had happened. I searched through information on the subject and found nothing that could explain why my sixth sense had suddenly dried up for no apparent reason.

Finally, while at Borders bookstore in San Francisco, I found a reference that gave me some hope. Although she had no explanation as to why, the author of a book on extra sensory perceptions told the story of how her own abilities had dried up for several years. She went on to share that when they did return they were stronger than ever. Heartened to learn that it wasn't unheard of and that there was a possibility they would return, I went back to trying to uncover what was leaving me feeling so horribly fatigued and ill.

In July 2009, I had the conversation with Aaron that would change my life; one that led me to discover remedies that alleviated the terrible symptoms which had been plaguing me for years.

Not long after I began wearing the bracelets, Aaron and I both noted that not only had my psi abilities returned; they were stronger than ever. Although this seemed to validate what I'd read in that book, I wanted a better answer. I wanted to know why.

◊ THIRTY TWO ◊

JAMMING THE FREQUENCY

YEARS ago, a couple of guys I worked with brought radio-controlled devices to work. One was a car and the other a dinosaur. Interestingly, because they utilized the same RF frequency, both could not operate at the same time. It was as if they canceled each other out. However, if only one was activated then the toy worked fine. I believe I was dealing with a similar situation.

All energy carries a unique frequency. Psi energy is no different, and my ability to function at a level of mind where I had access to the psi frequencies was compromised because the psi frequencies were blocked by EM waves of a different frequency. Once I was able to block those damaging EM frequencies by wearing the bracelets and the necklace, my ability to access the psi frequencies was restored. In fact, the more copper and silver I was exposed to, the stronger the psi abilities became.

While we were in Silver City, Nevada, I had a rather intriguing experience. Before getting out of the car to look around, I pointed to a large boulder and stated that it was a grave marker. I had never been to the former mining town so that itself was interesting. However, while I was standing at the marker, I remember looking to a place not far away from the boulder and feeling absolutely certain there was a grave there. There was no headstone and no other evidence this was true, but I still *knew* there was a grave. As I got into the car I shared this information with Aaron. He had witnessed enough displays of my psi abilities over the years to accept my declaration without even raising an eyebrow.

Once we returned home I got on the Internet. While I was primarily concerned with the mineral content of the area in and around Virginia City, Silver City, and Carson City, I was also very curious about the grave marker.

A plaque on the boulder read:

ILL-FATED BROTHERS
TWO WELL-EDUCATED BROTHERS, HOSEA AND
ETHAN GROSH, DISCOVERED SILVER
HERE IN 1856 BUT BOTH DIED IN 1857
BEFORE THEIR ORE WAS ASSAYED. HAD
THEY LIVED THEY MIGHT HAVE GONE ON
TO LOCATE THE COMSTOCK LODE.
THEIR CABIN WAS 1/4 - MILE TO THE SOUTH.

It had been in the direction of the cabin that I felt certain there had been another grave.

Researching further, I found an old newspaper article from the 19th century that referenced the marker and the site beyond it in-depth. I remember well how I felt when I read that a young squaw had been murdered and her body dumped into a well[37]. The well was located exactly where I told Aaron the other grave was.

It would seem that the mineral rich geology of Silver City definitely had a positive effect on my psi abilities.

There is both scientific and anecdotal documentation linking the use of a Faraday cage to increased psychic abilities. The Faraday cage blocks electromagnetic radiation just as the copper, silver, and zinc metals have done for me.

In the section on meditation I mentioned that my ability to meditate had been compromised by the EMFs. I knew that the EMFs were affecting my brain waves, keeping me from maintaining the alpha state associated with the Silva Method of meditation. However, it went deeper than that.

The Silva Method, developed by Jose Silva, teaches people to go to the alpha level which is a level of relaxation. The students are then taught how to solve problems while at this level of relaxation. A common side benefit from this method of meditation is achieving psychic ability. In point of fact, the final exercise during the Basic Lecture Series (BLS) demonstrates to students that they are able to do psychorientology. *This means educating the mind to function consciously within its own psychic dimension.*[38] Students use this ability to heal and solve problems at a distance, the intention being to make the world a better place.

I had been successfully using the Silva Method since graduating from the BLS in 2000. However, I had noticed that beginning in April 2008, I was not only unable to maintain levels of meditation, when I attempted to use the method to solve problems, I literally got the exact opposite of whatever I was trying to achieve. To say this was frustrating would be an understatement.

At one point I contacted senior lecturers of the Silva Method and obtained additional sound recordings designed to help an individual remain at the appropriate level of meditation. They also offered various suggestions aimed at helping me achieve the results I was working toward. However, in spite of extraordinary and focused effort, I was unable to correct the problem, and, right up until I left California, I achieved the exact opposite of whatever I tried to accomplish through the Silva Method. Interestingly, after a couple of months in my new home, I decided to try using the Silva Method again. In my new environment, away from the interference of EMFs, I found that I obtained successful results, consistently, and rather quickly. Additionally, I no longer had any difficulty maintaining deep levels of meditation.

Psychic ability is a phenomenon believed to be possessed by only a small percentage of people. Polls have shown that between 1.5 and 3 percent of the population have EMF Sensitivity; again, a rather small percentage. If one considers that psychics are able to sense things not detectable by the average individual, and that EMF sensitivities are able to sense electromagnetic energies not detectable by the average individual, then another relationship comes to light. I can't help but wonder if people who are EMF sensitive aren't also natural psychics.

◊ THIRTY THREE ◊

OLD PATTERNS THROUGH A NEW LENS

TO say the discovery of EMF Sensitivity has impacted my life would be a great understatement. Aside from the relief I gained, through research and trial and error I was able to make sense of events and health situations that had been puzzling me for years.

For example, ever since I was a teenager, in the hours and days prior to a thunderstorm I would experience excruciating migraines that often landed me in the emergency room. In fact, I could almost guarantee that I would be seeing the ER staff the last weekend of April and the first weekend in May, as this was the height of the Midwest thunderstorm season.

I sought out specialists and even spent time at a headache clinic, and while various theories were proposed, the cause of the migraines was never really established. What was worse, no medication ever alleviated the migraines. The stronger, narcotic type of drugs simply made the pain bearable and allowed me to sleep until the weather pattern moved on and the pain disappeared.

I learned through my research that extremely low frequencies associated with thunderstorms occur between the surface of the earth and its ionosphere. Suspecting that these frequencies were responsible for the terrible migraines I had suffered, I decided to see if the therapies I had found for the fault line EMFs would help with the migraines. Happily, I can say they do.

Beginning twelve to twenty-four hours before a storm system appears in our geography I would begin to feel symptoms similar to those I suffered near fault lines. In particular, I experienced a change in mood, a toothache, and pressure on my skull that would evolve into a migraine if I didn't intercede.

Taking the change in mood, usually a mild depression, as the first indication that a storm front was on its way, I put on the bracelets and necklace. Within a short time the symptoms alleviated. If there was any residual, I found that listening to the music from my therapy list finished them off.

Another revelation was seeing a relationship between past health issues and certain locales. In the past I did quite a bit of traveling for my job, and over the years I periodically experienced mysterious symptoms that were attributed to a variety of causes. Interestingly, medications prescribed at the time had been ineffective, puzzling my doctor. Recent research revealed that the locations where I felt the symptoms were on top of geologic fault zones. Additionally, comparative analysis confirmed that the symptoms were the same as those I was experiencing in the Bay Area.

A more amusing observation was my occasional reference to certain cities or geographic areas as being *a dump*. While studying fault line maps as part of my research, I noticed that without exception, the areas I had described as being dumps had geologic fault lines beneath them. At the time I visited these places I was completely unaware of my sensitivity to the EMFs emitted by fault lines. What made my colorful description so amusing, particularly to my husband, was that these very locations are considered some of the most affluent and desirable parts of our country.

I also learned that what is paradise for one person may not be for another. Case in point? Hawaii.

I have had the good fortune to visit the Hawaiian Islands more than once. They are incredibly beautiful; places I could easily relax. Maybe, too much since I lose all motivation to do anything else.

In fact, every time I have visited one of the islands I have made a point of stating that there was no way I could live in Hawaii.

"I would never get anything done."

My ability to think while in Hawaii was compromised, but since I was usually on vacation it didn't seem to be a problem. However, when I tried to take a working vacation there in 2008, I found I had a great deal of difficulty. For one thing, I was fatigued beyond belief. I went through an entire case of Diet Coke in less than two weeks, and that was in addition to the one and sometimes two lattes I was consuming each day. At the time I attributed it to stress and focused on the beautiful surroundings.

In hindsight, I realize that the electromagnetic frequencies emitted by Hawaii's unique geological features, including volcanoes and fault lines, were causing my problems.

◊ THIRTY FOUR ◊

ODDS AND ENDS

THE intent of writing this book was to share what I've learned in the hope that others who suffer from EMF Sensitivity will benefit from the information and be able to find relief from their symptoms. The following is anecdotal information based on my personal observations and experiences. It didn't really fit into any other part of the book and yet I believe the additional insight will be of benefit to others, so I have elected to include it in a separate section.

MAGNETS

For decades alternative practitioners have promoted the curative effects of magnets. Indeed, while working toward my doctorate I had a class in magnetic healing. However, my personal experience has been anything but positive. While small magnets, such as those we hang on the refrigerator, have no negative effect on me, the materials sold for therapeutic purposes cause me intense discomfort and, frequently, pain.

When in New Age stores I have to steer clear of baskets of hematite and other magnetic stones and recently, while speaking to someone selling magnetic jewelry at a metaphysical fair, I had to stand several feet away from her booth. At the time I was wearing the protective jewelry and still felt painful sensations. I caution readers to be sensitive to how various materials make you feel and to respond accordingly.

METAL SENSITIVITY

After years of trouble-free dental cleanings, I recently experienced a series of very unpleasant and painful jolts anytime the metal dental scaler touched my gum line. This included the metal tip of the instrument they were using to apply a numbing gel in order to proceed with the cleaning.

Interestingly, this is the first time in over ten years that a Cavitron© ultrasonic scaler has not been used. What makes it even more fascinating is that the Cavitron works by applying a high frequency oscillating magnetic field across a conductive metal stack, in which is induced a reactive magnetic field. The frequency is either 25,000 or 30,000 Hz. The mechanical vibrations produced are conveyed to a dental instrument that delivers a steady stream of water to the working tip.

Since I have never had difficulty before, I can only conclude that something about the magnetic field, if not the continuous use of water, precludes the metal instrument in the Cavitron from causing the same painful sensitivity that happens when using a traditional hand scaler. If someone is particularly sensitive during dental cleanings, it may be worth exploring the use of an ultrasonic scaler to see if there is a reduction in sensitivity.

CRYSTALS

I have not personally experienced any improvement from crystals or gemstones, but I encourage others to give them a try. A large selection can be found at your local New Age store. Although you can purchase online, I suggest you spend the time and energy physically touching the stones and crystals, determining which, if any, might help you feel better, and which ones you may want to avoid. Don't rely on the descriptions of what each stone or gem is reputed to do, go by how they make you feel. Keep in mind that what works for one person may not for another, so be your own judge.

HEAT

It was Aaron who first suggested that high temperatures may have an effect on my symptoms. He observed that I seemed to feel worse when out in the summer heat, which, in the East Bay, can easily see temperatures rise into triple digits Fahrenheit.

Preliminary observations suggested no relationship between heat and my symptoms. However, when I was in the mineral shop in Virginia City, in addition to having difficulty breathing, I felt inexplicably warm. I remember putting a hand to my head to see if I had a fever. When I left the shop this feeling eased, which is ironic because we were in the Nevada desert in August.

I later learned that one of the symptoms reported by those who are sensitive to EMFs was a feeling of warmth or a burning sensation similar to sunburn.

I continued to study the relationship between heat and how I felt and came to the following conclusions:

- Exposure to certain EMFs causes me to feel as if I have a fever.
- High temperatures will exacerbate the symptoms of EMF Sensitivity under certain circumstances

There is an exception to that last observation.

Exercise is one of the therapies I used to relieve symptoms. I noticed that when exposed to high temperatures, if I was participating in an activity that elevated my heart rate similar to doing cardio training, the symptoms were moderated.

AUTOMOBILES

While doing research on the Internet I came across an article that said the automobile was one of the worst places for someone with EMF Sensitivity. The author claimed that the electronic components in the car were responsible for the symptoms felt.

My personal experience has been the exact opposite. Other than when driving over fault lines, I have discovered that the steel and high metal content in the body and engine of the car actually provide a great deal of shielding. I recently noticed a definite difference in how I felt while in Boulder. For me, being in the car actually brings a level of symptomatic relief.

YAWNING

In a previous section I mentioned that one of the annoying and uncomfortable symptoms of EMF Sensitivity was excessive and abnormal yawning. I noted that there was a similarity to when I had been on an anti-seizure medication for a short time decades earlier.

Further investigation into yawning revealed that users of psilocybin mushrooms, also known as magic mushrooms, often described a marked stimulation of yawning while intoxicated, along with excess watering of the eyes and nasal mucous.[39]

While driving over fault lines, I not only had the excessive and often painful yawning, my eyes watered and burned, and I had a constantly runny nose.

Psilocybin enters the central nervous system and disrupts the serotonin levels in the brain. Serotonin is an important neurotransmitter. I found the similarities in yawning symptoms reported by users of the hallucinogenic drug, and the ones I suffered because of exposure to EMFs from fault lines, striking. It underscored the havoc the electromagnetic waves wreak on the brain.

FENG SHUI

Feng Shui translates to wind and water. It is an ancient Chinese system of aesthetics that uses the laws of astronomy and geography to help one improve their life in several areas including health. A long-time amateur practitioner of Feng Shui, I immediately noticed a similarity between the therapies I was using to treat symptoms of EMF Sensitivity and cures found in Feng Shui books and reference materials.

I noted that practitioners of this ancient art frequently mentioned dragon lines, referring to the energy meridians of the Earth. These were sometimes called Ley Lines. A great deal is written about the potential harm these meridians can cause and numerous steps to take to repel their damaging energies.

It may be worthwhile to integrate this practice into your overall plan of recovery. There are many excellent books that can help guide you.

PAU D'ARCO TEA

Even after I found the therapies that reduced or eliminated symptoms, my system continued to be affected. I was weak from years of exposure to problematic EMFs. I needed a way to boost my recovery, to regain my strength. The answer? For me, it was pau d'arco tea.

Also known as taheebo, it is a natural herb derived from the inner bark of the taheebo tree. It is has been used for centuries to treat a variety of ailments and to promote good health, and was used as a strengthening tonic by natives of South America. Within about a week of drinking two cups of pau d'arco tea each day I felt much stronger, and as if my body was well on its way to recovering its strength after the ordeal I had been living.

L-METHIONINE

Because of the confusion between SAMe and this amino acid, it is difficult to find accurate information about L-

Methionine. However, I can share that preliminary results in using it as a therapy have been incredibly positive. Within ten minutes of taking a dose, the symptoms from EMF Sensitivity are completely eliminated.

I worked with two different forms of the therapy. In one instance, I took capsules of L-Methionine along with a b-complex vitamin. In another, I stirred one tablespoon of Twin Labs' Amino Fuel in a small glass of water. In my own situation, I had the best results with a combination of the two. I recommend working with your health care provider to help you fine-tune the dose that works for you.

In a previous chapter I mentioned that during times of intense EMF Sensitivity, I craved margaritas and red wine. Just like L-Methionine, alcoholic beverages, and red wine in particular, have anti-inflammatory properties.

Note: *I strongly advise against using SAMe as a source of L-Methionine. It is a different compound and will be broken down differently in the body. Also, some individuals, including me, suffer nasty side effects from SAMe.*

Be sure to take a b-vitamin complex when taking L-Methionine. It helps the compound break down appropriately, and convert into either L-Methionine or L-cysteine, and not homocysteine, which can be harmful.

TRY A DIFFERENT DEVICE

While the majority of my symptoms are caused by Mother Nature's EMFs, I have found that I am also affected by certain manmade technologies. I have successfully used different approaches in different situations. In the case of the laser printer I elected to simply unplug it when not in use. However, in the case of the DVD player, I purchased a new one.

I advise people who find that their cell phones or other personal devices cause them problems to try swapping to another model. Another option is to quit using a wireless headset and see if a wired one makes a difference, or to use the speakerphone on the device and have it resting a distance away.

If you switched to a cordless phone at home, go back to using a wired one. It may be less convenient but it also may just do the trick. Experiment.

IT'S NOT YOUR WIRELESS — OR IS IT?

When I realized that something in my office was causing me difficulty I carefully considered everything that was in there, including the wireless. I was more than aware that this is number one on the hit parade for people critical of the rapid spread of technology.

Personally, I think it gets a bad rap and isn't responsible for even half of the complaints out there. What's more, I think all the negative press has created a kind of group hysteria that has brought about a *me too* situation where more people claim to be affected than actually are, or if they are, they are incorrectly assuming the source of the problem EMFs is wireless technology.

However, in light of what I learned through my own experience, I want to point out that the wireless device may be responsible for symptoms *but not because of the wireless frequencies emitted by the device.*

It may actually be that the wireless devices are but a few of the numerous electronic appliances plugged in at one location; more than likely all into the same power strip. In this case, it is the EMFs from the electrical draw and the overloaded power strip that are likely causing the problem, not the wireless frequencies. By relocating some of the devices to another location and redistributing the way the remaining appliances are plugged in, you are very likely to resolve any symptoms immediately.

IF YOU AREN'T USING IT; UNPLUG IT

Because so many of us depend on technology for our livelihood, it isn't practical to simply throw everything away, and pack up and move to a deserted island in the Pacific. Besides, if we are sensitive to Mother Nature's EMFs, it wouldn't do any good anyway.

In this case it makes sense to unplug anything not in use. Don't simply power it off; there is a slight draw of electrical current as long as something is plugged in. Go the next step and unplug it. It can make a huge and immediate difference.

OTHER COUNTRIES AND THEIR FREQUENCIES

When working in mobile and wireless technology in the early 1990s, I discovered that different regions of the world use different regulated radio frequencies. For example, in some European countries the part of the spectrum that the US has allocated for public use is for government use only.

Cell phones designed for US-only will not work in Europe. This is because they run on different wireless frequencies.

People who travel internationally may find that they have symptoms of EMF Sensitivity while using certain devices in one country but not necessarily while in another.

Interestingly, EMF Sensitivity is more widely accepted as a valid health condition in Europe.

◊ **THIRTY FIVE** ◊

LIVING WITH EMF SENSITIVITY

IN spite of the fact that the WHO and some European governments recognize EMF Sensitivity, skeptics and many professionals in the United States continue to dismiss it and propose that those who claim to be affected receive psychotherapy.

Ah, if only experience was transferrable.

The remedies I've discovered have enabled me to live a normal life and to interact with technology. However, because I am sensitive to certain electromagnetic frequencies I have to take definite steps to ensure that this remains so.

For instance, I have to wear the jewelry pretty much twenty-four hours a day, every day. I never know when I may find myself driving over a fault line or entering an environment that results in symptoms. The bracelets and necklace are my way of being proactive.

I keep Benadryl and chewing gum in the car in case the symptoms increase beyond what my jewelry is able to address.

Because exposure to fluorescent lighting for an extended length of time brings an intense difficulty concentrating, I have to make sure I am chewing gum before going into a retail establishment. If I don't, I can't remain in the store for more than about ten to twenty minutes before it becomes so bad I find myself feeling very spaced out and often forgetting what I went in for.

If I know the family is going to a location where fault lines are a strong likelihood, I have to bring a variety of remedies from my toolkit to ensure that I am able to diminish and/or eliminate what symptoms I can. For instance, during a recent trip to Las Vegas for a friend's wedding, we drove through Southern Utah, an area filled with geologic fault zones. In addition to the jewelry, I had to pull out my iPod in order to listen to the music choices I'd collected for times when the symptoms from EMF Sensitivity got bad.

I keep a journal of information and am constantly looking for opportunities to learn from research. I do not ever make assumptions about what is causing the symptoms and I do not see EMFs as being responsible for every little hiccup in my life. *Sometimes a cigar is just a cigar.*

I work hard to make sure that this condition does not take over my life.

Living with EMF Sensitivity has been one of the most difficult challenges I have had to deal with. The physical, mental, and emotional stress from years of unexplained symptoms that included debilitating fatigue was overwhelming. I had tried so many therapies with little to no success and suffered, helpless, as the symptoms grew in number and intensity at random and for no understandable reason. A number of times I thought I was losing my sanity or worried that I was dying and wouldn't live to see my kids grow up.

I know this has been especially hard on my family. No one wants to see someone they care for suffer. I hope that in sharing the personal impact of EMF Sensitivity, I am able to educate and perhaps inspire others who may be affected, to let them know that relief is possible.

Never give up.

About the Author

Elizabeth Maxim spent twenty years working as a consultant in the Information Technology industry. Her customer base included global Fortune 500 companies and she is a repeat speaker at industry conferences.

Elizabeth was raised with the belief that the best doctor is Mother Nature. She studied alternative medicine with an MD for several years before eventually earning a Doctor of Philosophy in this field. She also holds a bachelor's in holistic childcare.

NOTES

1 http://earthquake.usgs.gov/earthquakes/recenteqscanv/
2 Faraday cage. (2010, June 25). In *Wikipedia, The Free Encyclopedia*. Retrieved 17:57, June 26, 2010, from http://en.wikipedia.org/w/index.php?title=Faraday_cage&oldid=370064256
3 http://www.purestcolloids.com/history-copper.php
4 Fight-or-flight response. (2010, June 25). In *Wikipedia, The Free Encyclopedia*. Retrieved 18:08, June 26, 2010, from http://en.wikipedia.org/w/index.php?title=Fight-or-flight_response&oldid=370125782
5 http://www.nutros.net/nsr-02008.html
6 http://elizabethmaxim.com/projects/riding-the-waves/
7 http://www.stanford.edu/dept/news/pr/91/911231Arc1006.html
8 New Madrid Seismic Zone. (2010, June 3). In *Wikipedia, The Free Encyclopedia*. Retrieved 14:56, June 12, 2010, from http://en.wikipedia.org/w/index.php?title=New_Madrid_Seismic_Zone&oldid=365897440
9 http://earthquake.usgs.gov/hazards/qfaults/co/
10 http://www.ehso.com/fluorescent_safety.php
11 http://www.fcc.gov/
12 http://www.ieee.org/index.html
13 Electromagnetic hypersensitivity. (2010, June 10). In *Wikipedia, The Free Encyclopedia*. Retrieved 18:39, June 26, 2010, from http://en.wikipedia.org/w/index.php?title=Electromagnetic_hypersensitivity&oldid=367174055
14 Noise-cancelling headphones. (2010, June 25). In *Wikipedia, The Free Encyclopedia*. Retrieved 18:46, June 26, 2010, from http://en.wikipedia.org/w/index.php?title=Noise-cancelling_headphones&oldid=370007297
15 http://www.gi.alaska.edu/ScienceForum/ASF7/761.html
16 Sound. (2010, June 21). In *Wikipedia, The Free Encyclopedia*. Retrieved 18:51, June 26, 2010, from http://en.wikipedia.org/w/index.php?title=Sound&oldid=369269632

[17] http://www.gi.alaska.edu/ScienceForum/ASF7/761.html

[18] Histamine. (2010, June 22). In *Wikipedia, The Free Encyclopedia.* Retrieved 22:29, July 8, 2010, from http://en.wikipedia.org/w/index.php?title=Histamine&oldid=369564258

[19] Inflammation. (2010, July 5). In *Wikipedia, The Free Encyclopedia.* Retrieved 22:26, July 8, 2010, from http://en.wikipedia.org/w/index.php?title=Inflammation&oldid=371827893

[20] http://kids.nationalgeographic.com/kids/stories/spacescience/brain/

[21] Brainwave entrainment. (2010, June 15). In *Wikipedia, The Free Encyclopedia.* Retrieved 18:55, June 26, 2010, from http://en.wikipedia.org/w/index.php?title=Brainwave_entrainment&oldid=368180579

[22] http://josesilva.info/alpha_centering_sound.htm

[23] Pokémon episodes removed from rotation. (2010, June 22). In *Wikipedia, The Free Encyclopedia.* Retrieved 19:13, June 26, 2010, from http://en.wikipedia.org/w/index.php?title=Pok%C3%A9mon_episodes_removed_from_rotation&oldid=369638526

[24] Michael Persinger. (2010, June 15). In *Wikipedia, The Free Encyclopedia.* Retrieved 19:22, June 26, 2010, from http://en.wikipedia.org/w/index.php?title=Michael_Persinger&oldid=368117870

[25] http://www.scientificexploration.org/journal/jse_05_1_yoshino.pdf

[26] http://www.geotimes.org/feb07/WebExtra021507.html

[27] http://news.yahoo.com/s/space/20100609/sc_space/moreactivesunmeansnastysolarstormsahead

[28] DOE/Los Alamos National Laboratory (2008, January 3). Sound Waves Can Trigger Earthquake Aftershocks. *ScienceDaily.*

[29] http://www.aehf.com/articles/em_sensitive.html

[30] http://elizabethmaxim.com/2010/05/04/have-you-ever-seen-someone-eat-dirt/

[31] http://silvamethod.com/

[32] http://www.rps.psu.edu/probing/adhd.html

[33] Hynek Burda, Sabine Begall, Jaroslav Cerveny, Julia Neef, and Pavel Nemec. (2009, March 16). Extremely Low-frequency Electromagnetic

Fields Disrupt Magnetic Alignment of Ruminants. *Proceedings of the National Academy of Sciences, Vol. 106, No. 11.*

[34] Nicholls B, Racey PA, 2007 Bats Avoid Radar Installations: Could Electromagnetic Fields Deter Bats from Colliding with Wind Turbines?. PLoS ONE 2(3): e297. http://www.plosone.org/article/info%3Adoi%2F10.1371%2Fjournal.pone.0000297

[35] http://news.nationalgeographic.com/news/pf/79158083.html

[36] http://pinewooddesign.co.uk/2008/05/12/earthquake-cloud-prediction/

[37] Dan DeQuille [William Wright], *History of the Big Bonanza* (1877), pp. 1-46. http://www.nevadaobserver.com/Reading Room Documents/DeQuille 01 (1877).htm

[38] http://www.healthwithhypnosis.com/silva-method-of-mind-control/History of The Silva Method.htm

[39] Yawn. (2010, June 26). In *Wikipedia, The Free Encyclopedia.* Retrieved 01:56, June 27, 2010, from http://en.wikipedia.org/w/index.php?title=Yawn&oldid=370222048